It's All
Fogged Up

It's All Fogged Up

Zaeem Siddiqui

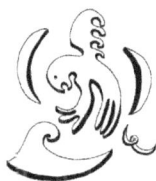

Life Rattle Press

It's All Fogged Up by Zaeem Siddiqui
Published in Canada by Life Rattle Press
Toronto, Ontario, Canada

Copyright © 2016 by Zaeem Siddiqui

ISBN 978-1-987936-22-3

Life Rattle Press New Publishers Series

Printed and bound in the United States

Contents

It's All
Fogged Up

" Write what disturbs you,
what you fear, what you
have not been willing to
speak about. Be willing to
be split open. "

- Natalie Goldberg

Chapter One

What's the Point?

Nine years. My name is Bob and I've been chronically depressed for nine years. Almost a decade. Every single day has been physically, emotionally, and mentally draining. I am exhausted. I don't eat, I can't sleep, and the world is nothing but grey.

When I was first diagnosed with chronic depression, I was pleased. I finally had a name to put to the awful feelings I had been experiencing for years. Depression. The word weighed heavy on my tongue. An innocuous ten letter word hiding the ineffable evil which would eventually contaminate every aspect of my life.

At the time, I didn't realise how big a deal it was. I was just happy that I finally knew why I felt the way I did. It was because I was broken. And if I was broken, then that meant I could be fixed. I was excited at the possibility of going back to being my normal self.

Fast-forward to now, and that hope has all but fizzled away into nothingness. All because of that simple ten letter word. Depression. It has woven itself so deeply into the fabric of my life that I can't even remember the person I was before I was depressed.

Depression sucks. I'm sure there are infinitely more articulate and eloquent ways to put it, but "depression sucks" just about sums it up. I am sick and tired of being sick and tired. I'm going to beat my depression or die trying. That's where this book comes in. "It's All Fogged Up" is the manifestation of my experience with chronic depression. With this book, I'm aiming for three things.

First of all, I hope that this book helps people. For people dealing with depression, I know what you're going through. I may not be going through the same experience, but I'm going through something similar. I know how depression isolates you from everyone else and alienates you from yourself.

I hope that you read (and enjoy) this book and find solace in the fact that you are not alone. Remember that you can beat depression. If I can provide just one depressed person a sense of hope, a little ray of sunlight breaking through the all-encompassing fog that is depression, then I'll have done what I set out to accomplish.

For people who are not dealing with depression but want to learn more about it, I hope this book gives you insight into the mental illness. The chapters of this book were written during different periods of my depression. Some of them might be morbid and dark while others are annoyingly optimistic and motivational. An idea in one chapter might contradict one in another. Depression fluctuates a lot and I hope my writing encapsulates its many different forms.

The second thing I want to do with this book is reduce the negative stereotypes surrounding mental illnesses. I want this book to be relatively funny (hilarious would be pushing it), but more importantly, I want it to be informative. We avoid discussing mental health because we don't fully understand it. With this book, I hope to remedy this.

And I'm not doing it by myself; you're helping me mitigate stigma right now. By reading this book in public and discussing it with your friends, you will be raising awareness about mental health. We need more people like you in the world. Continue being awesome.

Together, you and I can create a social environment where people won't feel judged or ashamed of seeking the help they need. Discussing mental health can be awkward and uncomfortable, but that doesn't mean we should forego the conversation entirely.

Thirdly, I'm writing this book for myself. Writing externalises my thoughts and helps me sift through and organise them. It helps me vent. It is remarkably cathartic and therapeutic. At times, my writing may come across as a bit of a rant, and that's probably because I'm ranting. A lot of things annoy me.

Like wet socks, for example. Or people who chew with their mouths open. Or those stupid fake pockets on t-shirts. Or people who walk really slowly for no reason at all. Or continuity errors in any movie or TV show. Or those five crucial seconds when your tea goes from boiling hot to ice-cold and undrinkable. Surprisingly, I don't mind Mondays. It's Tuesday I've got issues with. But, I digress.

The last thing I want to say is this: do not let the scientific jargon, philosophical ideas, clunky/mixed metaphors, and unnecessarily long-winded sentences fool you; I am not an expert on anything at all. I am just a fogged up guy with a laptop.

Of course, that doesn't mean I'm a *complete* moron (there are parts missing). I have done weeks of research to ensure that all the information I provide in this book is factually accurate. I've included insights from a wide spectrum of people who have suffered from one of the many forms of depression at some point in their lives. Most importantly, I've tried to ensure that everything I write in this book is at least mildly interesting.

If you feel that I've made an error somewhere in this book, please buy a fountain pen and blue ink, take some calligraphy classes, compose a beautiful and eloquent hand-written letter, proofread it, sign it, wait for the ink to dry, buy an envelope, put the letter in the envelope, seal it, and then keep it to yourself. Shame on you for trying to destroy what little self-esteem I have left. (Seriously though, just send me an email and we'll work it out.)

So why exactly am I writing this book?

Because depression doesn't get to win.

66 Maybe you have to know the darkness before you can appreciate the light. "

- Madeleine L'Engle

- Chapter Two -

The F-Bomb

What is depression? It's a simple question to ask, but impossible to answer properly. There are many ways to talk about depression. You could shout, whisper, mutter, or sing, for example. OK, I admit, that joke was beyond awful. I'm sorry. To be fair, I did warn you that my jokes are terrible and cringeworthy.

On a more serious note, the two most common ways to explain depression are by listing a bunch of symptoms and hoping you'll get the gist of the experience, or by going over the physical aspects of depression and explaining what it does to your brain. I prefer a slightly different method, where I explain depression through an unnecessarily convoluted and drawn-out analogy which sounds good on the surface, but is overused throughout the book and ends up making less of an impact than I had hoped it would.

But before we get to my excellent analogy, let's address the most irritating thing people think about depression. Although society is becoming more aware about the importance of mental health, there are still many people who cling to the view that depression is just being sad for a really long time. Worse still, these people think being depressed is intentional.

They think depression is like a video game which you can stop playing whenever you want, but you actively decide to keep on playing because you enjoy it or because you want the attention, or because of some equally trivial reason. To top it off, these people are so arrogant in their ignorance that they have the audacity to tell you to "snap out of it". They think they're pointing to some kind of massive OFF button for your depression and all you need to do is press it.

*I've been feeling like an absolute waste of a human being for nine years and you're telling me I could have stopped whenever I wanted? "Just snap out of it," huh? That's amazing advice! I hadn't even considered it in the nine years I've been suffering from depression! Let me try it right now! *Snaps out of it* Done! Now I can* *live my life like a healthy functioning member of society! Thank you, kind stranger, for your profound insight into my medical condition has cured me of my depression completely! Go forth and share your infinite wisdom with the rest of the world!*

If only it were that simple. Brace yourself, dear reader, because I'm about to drop an F-bomb on your face. That stands for 'Fact Bomb', by the way. All the kids are using it these days. The idea is simple; I will bombard you with so many facts that you will eventually break down and cower before my intellectual superiority.

Of course, this strategy works best when using uppercase letters. Obviously, the bigger my letters are, the smarter and more factually accurate I must be. That being said, I'm against CAPITAL punishment, so I'll just write like I normally do.

Depression is not a choice. Depression is not something which only affects emotionally underequipped people. Depression can affect anyone, regardless of age, gender, socioeconomic status, intellectual acuity, or location. Depression doesn't care about who you are.

Depression affects more than 350 million people worldwide and it is estimated that by the year 2030, depression will be the second-highest medical cause of disability. Roughly 11% of adolescents will experience a depressive disorder by the age of 18. Close to 55% of people suffering from depression don't even realise that they're depressed! Worse, 58% of people over the age of 65 think that depression is normal by their age.

But these are just numbers. Numbers don't explain what depression does to you. People say depression is "a chemical imbalance in the brain" but that doesn't explain anything either. Reducing something to its physical attributes doesn't explain anything. It's like saying the Eiffel Tower is a metal structure. Technically, you're not wrong. But there's so much more to it than that.

So instead of looking at statistics, let's talk about how depression physically changes the brain. A study done by the University of Sydney's Brain and Mind Research Institute, published in *Molecular Psychiatry*, found that people who suffer from chronic depression have a smaller hippocampus than those who have never experienced depression. The hippocampus is the part of the brain which is in charge of memory, learning, and emotion. Partnered with the amygdala, the emotional centre of the brain, the hippocampus helps turn our short-term memory to our long-term memory.

The hippocampus connects emotions and senses to our memories before it stores them. If you think of a moment which made you happy, like when you bought this book, the hippocampus comes into play. It will associate the feeling of happiness with the smell of a new book or the feeling of the pages beneath your fingers, and then it will store that memory in your brain.

When you are suffering from depression, the hippocampus shrinks. (If you want to sound clever when you tell people about this, the scientific term for this brain shrinkage is *hippocampal atrophy*.) Compared to a healthy brain, the brain of a person suffering from depression is much smaller than normal; in some cases, the hippocampus can shrink to 80% of its original volume! The longer you are depressed, the more the neurons in your hippocampus deteriorate, and the smaller your hippocampus becomes.

This means that it becomes harder for you to form new memories. It also means that you lose the ability to efficiently recall memories which are stored in your long-term memory. Think of your long-term memory like a gigantic filing cabinet. Each memory is a file in a folder in this filing cabinet. Your hippocampus (along with the other parts of the brain involved in this process) is the personal assistant who kindly files everything without uttering threats under her breath.

Every time you remember something, your hippocampus goes into the filing cabinet, finds the right folder, and picks out the file you wanted. All the files in this filing cabinet are linked in some way. For example, the file for "Hammer" might be linked to multiple files. It could be linked to the file for "Thor", the file for "Time", and the file for "Things I Gave To My Neighbour But Never Got Back".

You might not always understand how these files are linked, but you don't need to. That's what your hippocampus is for. Whenever a new memory is created, the hippocampus will attach an emotion or feeling to that memory and then go to the filing cabinet and store it in the right location. It does all of this incredibly quickly.

The more often you remember a particular thing, the quicker the hippocampus retrieves the file, because it knows where to look. But when you're depressed, your hippocampus 'forgets' where each file is. The filing system gets fogged up and your hippocampus loses the connections between files. It has to work a lot harder to find everything. You end up struggling to remember things properly and your brain finds it harder to create new memories because its personal assistant isn't as efficient as usual.

The good news is that hippocampal atrophy is reversible. The hippocampus regularly regenerates neurons and fixes the connections between cells, through a process known as neurogenesis. Serotonin, the neurotransmitter in your body responsible for happiness, mediates the regeneration of brain cells. Although the hippocampus is capable of neurogenesis by itself, sometimes it needs backup. This is why most antidepressants contain serotonin, because it is meant to kickstart neurogenesis in the hippocampus.

I'm shoving all these statistical, biological, and chemical facts in your face because it is important to remember that depression is a serious mental health condition. It should be treated as such. By telling a depressed person that it's as easy as "snapping out of it", what you're doing (from their perspective), is confirming their belief that they're just too weak to deal with something as trivial as feeling sad.

Such ignorance not only isolates depressed people more than the mental illness itself does, but it convinces them they're not strong enough to beat depression. Telling someone to "snap out of it" is not productive or helpful. It's not even worth the time it takes to say.

If you've no idea how to talk to someone dealing with a mental illness, don't feel bad. It's an awkward situation for both parties involved. But that doesn't mean you should avoid the conversation. Feel free to skip ahead to the last chapter of this book. **Could You Not?** I can't guarantee that what worked for me will be applicable to your situation, but hopefully it'll help you in some way.

As I mentioned in the previous chapter, one of the reasons I'm writing this book is to get rid of the negative stereotypes associated with depression and other mental illnesses. I'm writing it because I want to "defog" the mystery of depression. As you can probably tell by the title of the book and my oh-so-subtle quotation marks in the previous sentence, I think depression takes a very specific form.

Ten points to whomever can guess what it is.

SOURCES

"Depression Facts and Statistics." Fairfax Mental Health. www.fairfaxmentalhealth.com/depression-treatment.

(1992). The changing rate of major depression. Cross-national comparisons. Cross-National Collaborative Group. *JAMA*, 21, 3098–3105.

Czéh, B., Michaelis, T., et al. (2001). Stress-induced changes in cerebral metabolites, hippocampal volume, and cell proliferation are prevented by antidepressant treatment with tianeptine. *Proceedings of the National Academy of Sciences of the United States of America* 22, 12796–12801.

Mahar, I., Bambico, F. R., et al. (2013). Stress, serotonin, and hippocampal neurogenesis in relation to depression and antidepressant effects. *Neuroscience and Biobehavioral Reviews*, 173–192.

Sahay, A., & Hen, R. (2007). Adult hippocampal neurogenesis in depression. *Nature Neuroscience*, 9, 1110–1115.

Sapolsky, Robert M. (2001). Depression, antidepressants, and the shrinking hippocampus. *Proceedings of the National Academy of Sciences of the United States of America*, 98, 12320-12322. DOI: 10.1073/pnas.231475998.

Schmaal L, Veltman D, et al. (2015). Subcortical brain alterations in major depressive disorder: findings from the ENIGMA Major Depressive Disorder working group. *Molecular Psychiatry*. DOI: 10.1038/mp.2015.69

The National Institute for Health Care Management Research and Educational Foundation . "Improving Early Identification & Treatment of Adolescent Depression: Considerations & Strategies for Health Plans." NIHCM Foundation. www.nihcm.org/pdf/Adol_MH_Issue_Brief_FINAL.pdf

World Health Organization . "Depression." WHO. www.who.int/mediacentre/factsheets/fs369/en.

World Health Organization. "Global burden of mental disorders and the need for a comprehensive, coordinated response from health and social sectors at the country level." WHO International. apps who.int/gb/ebwha/pdf_files/EB130/B130_9-en.pdf

" Life is one long process of getting tired. "

- Samuel Butler

Chapter Three

Fogged Up

Depression is an all-encompassing fog that fills up my mind. It is dense and impenetrable, yet it isn't solid. If it were solid, I'd be able to punch it until my hands started bleeding. I'd be able to fight it. But my depression is vague and hazy and elusive. Its abstract nature makes it infinitely more sinister than a corporeal manifestation.

This fogged up mental illness pervades every aspect of my life and establishes itself in ways I can't even fathom. With a physical injury, doctors know exactly where to look, what to fix, and how to fix it. With depression, it's not as clear-cut. I can't point to a spot on my head and say that's where depression is. It's not all in my head anyway, because depression causes physical aches and pains all over my body.

Depression weighs me down. The fog is so dense that my actions are pointlessly slowed down, like I'm dragging a boulder and wading through quicksand. All of my movements are rough and spasmodic. Something as effortless as walking is no longer a fluid motion, but clumsy and disjointed. Even my thoughts become fragmented and erratic.

My perception of time is distorted, like I'm experiencing it in slow motion. By that, I mean it's not like that awesome Quicksilver scene in X-Men: Days of Future Past. It's more like I've been transformed into a sloth. Everyone else is getting on with their lives at a normal pace while I'm trapped in time. I am stuck inside my own head.

Depression also slows me down mentally. I can't tell you how much this frustrates me. The smallest of steps becomes a mountain which takes me days to climb. I can't speak in full sentences because my train of thought always gets lost in the fog. I've got so many thoughts competing for a megaphone, viciously fighting for the chance to be voiced, that my mouth can't figure out which one to say.

I'll start a sentence without knowing how it's supposed to end. My speech is full of pregnant pauses, awkward silences, and inane filler words because my brain is constantly struggling to catch up with the conversation. I am experiencing real-world lag. I can actually feel myself getting stupider. This causes me unimaginable stress.

I hate myself for being so useless that I can't speak like a normal human being. Is it too much to ask that I be able to construct a complete sentence? What the hell is wrong with me? I feel bad for making the person I'm talking to feel awkward. They usually just pretend that everything is fine because they don't know how else to deal with the situation. In some cases, they end up being way too nice to me because they pity my idiocy.

I keep verbal interactions to a minimum because I don't want to embarrass myself. People think I'm shy, but I'm just being careful. I've perfected the art of holding entire conversations without uttering a single word. I can just exhale through my nose, roll my eyes, raise my eyebrows, or make a random facial expression and people will instantly understand what I mean.

Talking to people comes bundled with the social custom of having to reply instantly. If you don't reply instantly (or within a couple of seconds), you come across as rude, uninterested in the conversation/person you're talking to, or just plain slow. Nobody enjoys talking to a person who can't keep up with the conversation.

That's why I prefer texting or chatting online. It's socially acceptable for me not to reply instantly during a textual conversation. In fact, it can even give the illusion that my social life is so active that I'm talking to multiple people at the same time. It can make people think I was too busy with other conversations to reply instantly.

Of course, the people who text me actually know the kind of person I am in real life, so they labour under no such delusion. They know I'm not replying because I feel I have nothing valuable to say. I suppose that's a benefit of my depression; it forces me to collect and critique my thoughts before I share them with others. When it's a textual conversation, I have all the time I need to formulate and edit my thoughts before I type them out. It's less awkward for all parties involved.

Depression fogs up my brain so much that I find it impossible to focus or stay productive. Let's say I want to make a nice hot cup of tea. I'll try to focus on that task while my depression will push all kinds of intrusive thoughts into my head. It'll add thoughts about how little I matter to the rest of the world, thoughts about how stupid I am, thoughts about how pointless my life is, thoughts about how I'm a complete failure, thoughts about how the world would be better off if I just kill myself. You know, the usual stuff.

As you can probably imagine, it's difficult to concentrate on something as trivial as tea when you're preoccupied with the futility of human existence. Fifteen minutes later, I'll still be standing in the same spot, staring intently at the little teabag floating aimlessly in the now-cold murky water. I'll feel terrible for wasting a perfectly good teabag as well as fifteen minutes of my life. My depression will convince me that my punishment for being so pathetic is to drink the liquid disgrace (to call it tea would be an insult to actual tea) and then continue feeling awful for how badly I've ruined my life (and that teabag).

The fog is disorienting. It isolates me and cuts me off from the rest of the world. I feel disconnected and alienated from everyone, even with I'm surrounded by my friends or family. I feel like I'm intruding on other people's lives just by existing. I need to apologise for being alive.

Depression covers my vibrant, colourful, and friendly world with an impenetrable layer of apathy. It transforms my world into a colourless vacuum, devoid of purpose and meaning. The fog is everywhere at once. Whatever it touches loses its value.

Eating, for example, no longer involves sensations like taste, or thoughts of how delicious the food is, or wondering how much more I'm going to eat later. Instead, it's just a mechanical process of chewing, swallowing, and digesting. That's it. No emotions. No taste. No desire. No satisfaction.

Eating is reduced to a series of motions my body goes through to ensure I don't starve. My depression takes away the enjoyment of food. It tells me that there are starving children all over the globe, so I have no right to eat. My depression tells me I am the walking embodiment of gluttony. When it's happy with my level of self-loathing, my depression forces me to eat. I feel awful for every bite I take, even if it's barely enough to keep me alive.

Depression is deceiving. The thick layer of fog masks sounds and shadows. I think I'm hallucinating. I see things which aren't really there. Random flutters of movement in the corners of my eyes. Voices whispering my name. Things disappearing from where I left them. An overwhelming suspicion that I'm being watched.

I'm constantly paranoid that people want to embarrass and humiliate me, even though the rational part of my mind knows this isn't true. I walk into a room, see someone smiling, and become convinced that he's smiling at a joke made at my expense. My depression tells me that the whole world is in on the joke apart from me. It's like I'm trapped in a situation like The Truman Show.

I'm unable commit to anything because I'm always waiting for something bad to happen. If a person does something nice for me, I will not be able to appreciate the gesture because I'll be too busy waiting for the impending disaster which must eventually follow. I'm waiting for the cameras to show up and the person to say "Surprise! It was all fake! Your entire life was a lie constructed just to entertain the rest of the world! Your failures amuse us!"

I know that the fear is stupid. It's totally irrational and illogical, but my fogged up mind has trouble seeing logic. In fact, my mind is so messed up that I have trouble seeing things which actually *are* there.

If your mind is free of fog, you see everything. You see your hopes, your dreams, your desires, your ambitions, your motivations; your future. You have a reason to keep on living. Your mind is clear and focused. Even if you don't know 100% what you want to do in life, you still have a vague idea of which direction you want go in.

Depression has stolen that visibility from me. It has clouded my judgement and blocked out everything. My mind is so foggy, I no longer see the point of living. I'm constantly tired, I barely sleep, and I don't eat. I have no energy, no drive, no ambitions, no desires, no hopes, no dreams.

It feels like I'm not really living. I'm dead and am just waiting to be buried. I'm pretending to be alive. I'm here because of existential inertia; I was forced into existence and I will continue to exist until the effects of that force dissipate and I can finally rest in peace.

Depression relentlessly berates and insults me. It disguises itself as my inner-voice so I can never tell if the thoughts in my head belong to me or my depression. I'm getting better at telling the difference now, though it's not always easy.

My depression finds the insecurities I've been hiding from the world and it shines a spotlight on them. It finds the doubts that whisper to me in the back of my mind and it hands each of them a megaphone. It finds the prison where I've locked away my fears and it lets them all out. It takes my self-confidence, straps it to a chair, and forces it to replay all the worst moments of my life on repeat until it breaks down completely.

Depression changes a person on a foundational level. Like a stubborn ninety year old with a juice box, depression sucks out everything, one laboured breath at a time.

It doesn't stop until you're empty and hollow. It strips you of the things which make you who you are. It takes everything from you until you are nothing but a feeble imitation of your former self.

Then depression sits inside your hollowed shell and takes over. It becomes you. And you become it. My depression and I are two halves of an incomplete idiot. Depression inserts itself into your life. It fills the crevices of your brain. It corrupts your personality. It infects your thoughts. It alienates you from yourself. It is an inescapable emptiness which somehow manages to fill you up.

Then depression plays its cruellest trick. It convinces you that it doesn't exist. My greatest fear is that I might not be depressed. I worry that I was misdiagnosed. What if this is who I actually am? The thought eats away at me. What if I genuinely am an apathetic, lethargic, self-centred, chronically insecure, pessimistic, pitiful, ungrateful, whiny excuse for a human being?

I'm terrified of looking in the mirror and seeing a non-depressed version of myself. As much as I hate depression, I want it. I *need it*. It's a symbiotic relationship. Depression is my security blanket. It is my scapegoat. I can hide behind it. It's the thing I can blame for me being the way I am.

Depression is a part of me. I feel like it's my defining characteristic. Without it, I wouldn't really be who I am. I wouldn't be me. A ring is defined by the absence of space in its centre. Without that hole, a ring is just a flat metal disk. In the same way, the inescapable emptiness of depression defines me. The emptiness envelopes me. It moulded me into the person I am today.

I don't necessarily *want* to be the sort of person that I am, but it's too late. I've come too far to be anything else. My depression is all I have left now and I hate it. I hate myself.

The scariest thing about depression is that you never really catch it fogging up your life. I tried once. I *mist*. (I'm not apologising for that joke). Depression sneaks its way into your life. You never see it coming. You just realise one day that you have no idea where you are or how you got there. By then, it's too late.

You're already lost in the fog.

66 May it be a light to you
in dark places, when all
other lights go out. **"**

- J.R.R. Tolkien,
The Fellowship of the Ring

- Chapter Four -

Dirty Laundry

One of the simplest truths of life is that things are scarier in the dark. We don't fear the dark itself. We're afraid of the things which hide inside it. We fear what we can't see. We fear what we can't understand. We are afraid of the unknown. This is evident in everyday life.

During the day, things are fine. The pile of clothes on your chair is just the pile of dirty laundry you swore you'd clean up three weeks ago. The quilt on your bed is just the thing you cover yourself with (and stick one foot out from under) when you're sleeping. The scraping sound is just the tree branch hitting your window whenever the wind blows. The hiss coming from underneath your bed is just the air conditioning turning on. Apart from the dirty laundry, these things aren't all that scary. But come nightfall, things change.

When it's dark, your brain goes on high alert. It becomes convinced that the pile of clothes on your chair is a monster, seconds away from butchering you and your family. Your shapeless quilt suddenly begins to look very much like a decaying body lying motionless on your bed; you can even hear the blood dripping down your footboard. The scraping sound is a demon child trying to claw its way through the window. The hiss under your bed is a gigantic snake slithering its way up through the springs in your mattress.

You peer into the darkness and you see eyes glaring back out at you. You hear whispers all around. You see indistinguishable figures moving around in the darkness. You jump at the slightest noise. Your brain is adamant that you're in danger. It freaks out. It panics. Rational thoughts are drowned out by the alarms blaring in your head. Things are a lot scarier in the dark.

In the world of mental health, this darkness is stigma. This negative stereotype makes mental illnesses seem scarier than they actually are. We acknowledge that it's a problem, but we're not doing enough to get rid of it. Society is a terrified four year old with his eyes clamped shut and his security blanket gripped tight, hoping against hope that the darkness will disappear before he has to open his eyes again.

Stigma is not a problem which will solve itself. We no longer have the luxury of being afraid of the dark. We have to stop hoping someone else will come along and turn the lights on for us. We need to turn on the lights ourselves.

Stigma about mental health and illness isn't a new thing. Like an unwelcome guest, it's been around for ages and shows no signs of leaving any time soon. We all know about lobotomies. This practice, which won a Nobel Prize, looked to alleviate suffering by cutting the brain's connection to the prefrontal cortex, the part of the brain where it was thought that mental illnesses originated. Not the best solution, I admit, but it did pave the way for bright sparks to link mental illnesses with neurological responses in the brain.

Trephination had the same idea (that's the one where they drill a hole through your head). The 18th century took a more physical approach to 'curing' mentally ill patients. Physicians had not yet figured out that physical and mental illnesses were different things. They thought that the same remedy could cure physical and mental illnesses at the same time. They resorted to ice baths, restraints, and forced isolation as potential cures to mental illnesses.

Physicians and religious folk also debated the logic of mental illnesses. Before even trying to cure the illness, many believed that depressed, schizophrenic, and bipolar individuals were possessed. They were convinced that mentally ill people needed exorcisms to be rescued from their inner demons. Then, the physical therapy could begin.

All of these treatments were a result of people's ignorance about mental health. They didn't understand what the problem was, so they tried to solve it using the only methods they knew. Even though we now know more about mental health than we did fifty years ago, we're still forced to deal with widespread ignorance and discrimination.

Like depression, this stigma has different forms. For example, it might be apparent in the fact that mental illnesses don't get the same insurance coverage as physical illnesses or it might be apparent in the fact that some people believe mental illnesses are intentional cries for attention. Stigma isn't always obvious and easy to identify.

What is obvious is that stigma, whether it's intentional or unintentional, is caused by ignorance. Many of us don't fully understand what mental illnesses are or how they affect people. We're afraid of people who suffer from mental illnesses.

The media isn't helping in any way at all. In any given news story, a person with mental health issues is depicted as being a dangerous, violent, mass murdering psychopath. Horrific acts committed by people suffering from a mental illness are sensationalized in the media simply because these kinds of stories will become viral.

Our opinions are influenced by what we see in the media. If all you see in the news is about how a mentally unstable person took down an airplane or how a mentally ill person shot up a school full of kids, *of course* you're going to be afraid of people suffering from mental illnesses.

The truth is that mental illnesses don't make people violent or likely to commit mass murders any more than a mentally healthy person. A person suffering from a mental illness is actually more likely be a victim of crime; not the perpetrator. We're too quick to link violence with terrorism or mental illness. This ignorance causes other problems, too.

People who suffer from mental illnesses will learn to hide their illness because they're afraid of being ostracized and judged by others. They're afraid of getting the help they need because of the social environment we've created. It's a circle of fear which helps no one and harms everyone.

We're trying to mitigate stigma, but it's our fault this stigma exists in the first place. Our ignorance, prejudice, and judgemental nature is preventing people from openly discussing mental health. We blame society, but we are society.

Of course, I don't mean to say that *everyone* is making matters worse. There are thousands of people trying their utmost best to learn more about mental illnesses and help get rid of stigma forever. Thanks to scientific advancements, we've come a long way from when our best idea was to drill a hole through a guy's head and hope that it solved everything. But we're not in the light just yet.

That's why I'm writing this book. I want to help turn the lights on. Permanently. I want to show people that mental illnesses aren't as scary as they seem. I want to show that people suffering from mental illnesses aren't people we should be terrified of. I want to shed light on this issue.

Obviously, my book isn't amazing or particularly well-written, so it's not like I've got a sun-like source pointed at stigma and discrimination. If anything, I've got a flickering candle. But even the dimmest light can illuminate a room, even if it's for the most fleeting of moments.

If we get rid of the darkness, the psychotic monster hell-bent on murdering you and your entire family is reduced to a pile of dirty laundry. Sure, that pile of dirty laundry is scary in its own right, but it's not as scary as we thought it was when the lights were off. It's still a problem, but it's manageable now. We can solve it if we learn to work together. We can solve it if we get rid of the darkness.

All we need to do is turn on the light.

" We're all in the same game, just different levels. Dealing with the same hell, just different devils. "

- Jason Phillips (Jadakiss)

Chapter Five

The Many-Faced Demon

The first step to turning on the lights is understanding depression. In a previous chapter, I talked about what *my* depression is like. The fog is my own experience of the mental illness. Other people will experience depression very differently.

A friend of mine described depression as being a ghost trapped in the world of the living. Another described it as an impossibly heavy weight on his chest. One person described it as being stuck in a hole she couldn't climb out of. There are so many ways to talk about depression because of how vague it is. It manifests itself in different ways, many of which are not always obvious.

One reason depression is misunderstood by so many is that we tend to use 'depression' as an umbrella term to talk about all the different types of this mental illness.

Even people who are suffering from depression don't always realise that there are multiple forms of depression. I've listed the five most common forms of depression below, but there are dozens more.

1. MAJOR DEPRESSIVE DISORDER

First up, we've got Major Depressive Disorder, which is also referred to as Major Depression. If you can't tell by the subtle name, this is a big deal. It is arguably the most common form of depression. That being said, not just any depression can be diagnosed as Major Depression; there are criteria you need to meet.

First of all, you need to have exhibited at least five symptoms from the list of symptoms published in the *Diagnostic and Statistical Manual of Mental Disorders (DSM)* by The American Psychiatric Association. The list includes symptoms such as fatigue, excessive guilt, anhedonia, suicidal thoughts, insomnia, and restlessness. Secondly, these symptoms (one of which has to be anhedonia) need to have persisted every single day for at least two weeks. Thirdly, these symptoms must have been so severe that they prevented you from functioning normally. Major Depression doesn't just slow you down, it flat-out stops you from living.

2. PERSISTENT DEPRESSIVE DISORDER (PDD)

Women are three times more likely to suffer from PDD than men. No, not the rapper. Well, maybe. I don't know. Anyway, PDD is a less severe kind of depression and is often referred to as chronic depression or dysthymia.

Its symptoms can also be found in the DSM. It has fewer symptoms than Major Depression but tends to last longer. Typically, the symptoms persist for at least two years. Unlike Major Depression, PDD isn't always constant either, its symptoms can disappear for weeks at a time. That being said, it's unlikely that you'd be able to go two months without experiencing any symptoms of PDD.

PDD doesn't stop you like Major Depression, but it slows you down considerably. What's worse is that you can have episodes of Major Depression while going through chronic depression. This is known as a 'Double Depression'. If PDD is like being forced to do an endless series of push-ups, then Double Depression is like doing push-ups with a sumo wrestler sitting on your back while someone stabs the inside of your elbows with a knife covered in lemon juice.

3. <u>Post-Partum Depression</u>

Giving birth throws your hormones into a frenzy, which can cause mood swings, anxiety, anhedonia, and insomnia. If these symptoms persist for more than two weeks, you could be experiencing Post-Partum Depression. Post-Partum Depression, as the name suggests, is a form of depression women may experience after giving birth.

It is not always obvious that a person is suffering from Post-Partum Depression, since the symptoms can reveal themselves months after child-birth. The symptoms are the same as those for PDD, but also include having problems emotionally connecting with the baby, feeling guilty for being a terrible mother, and thoughts of physically harming the baby. If it's still not clear, this form of depression only applies to women.

4. SEASONAL AFFECTIVE DISORDER (SAD)

People often conflate depression with sadness. They are completely different things. Obviously, the best way to stop people doing this is to come up with name for a depressive condition which can be abbreviated to "SAD". That'll teach those pesky people that depression and sadness are not the same thing.

Seasonal Affective Disorder is a type of depression which typically affects a person only during the winter months. It is dormant during the rest of the year. This depression has the same symptoms as PDD and is thought to be a result of lower exposure to sunlight compared to the summer months.

5. BIPOLAR DISORDER

Bipolar Disorder was previously known as Manic Depression. It is a mood disorder characterised by rapid swings between overly happy highs (mania) and extreme lows (depression). Symptoms of depressive episodes are the same as Major Depression, while the symptoms of manic episodes include rapid thoughts, increased energy, euphoria, and delusions of grandeur.

People suffering from Bipolar Disorder randomly shift between the two states of being. The shifts can be sudden or gradual. In most cases, a person suffering from Bipolar Disorder won't notice the change themselves. It's like sitting in a room while someone lowers the temperature by one degree every fifteen minutes.

These are just five different types of depression. Generalising the different forms of depression by using an umbrella term does very little to reduce the stigma surrounding mental illnesses. It demeans the struggles people suffering from depression are going through.

Because depression affects people so differently, it is impossible to make sweeping statements and come up with universal diagnoses or solutions. Doing so is dangerous and misinforms the public. Raising awareness about mental health is important but doing it the wrong way ends up enforcing the very stigma we're trying to get rid of in the first place.

Generalisations make people suffering from depression doubt their depression's existence. I cannot stress how unhelpful and risky this is. It effectively silences hundreds of people who are suffering from depression but aren't quite sure if they're depressed.

Furthermore, if you generalise the illness, you generalise the cure. Depressed people will feel worthless for not being able to cure themselves of depression using the 'universal' cure. They will think it's because they are too weak or stupid. They will blame themselves, even though it's not their fault.

I know this because I went through the same thing. I felt insignificant and helpless. People kept throwing pointless platitudes at me, telling me I could beat depression if I just exercised more or took a bunch of pills or stopped being so negative all the time. I tried what they suggested. It didn't work.

At the time, I didn't realise that depression is infinitely more intricate than we assume it to be. I thought the reason the 'cure' didn't work was because I must have been doing something wrong. My depression used this thought to take me on a guilt trip. My depression punished me for not being able to cure myself of it. Everyone else apparently cured themselves. Why couldn't I? My depression told me I deserved to be depressed. I couldn't think of a good enough reason to argue against it.

We need to explain that depression is unique to each individual. It cannot be generalised. It should not be generalised. It is a demon with many faces, many of which we have yet to see. And if you insist on talking about generic symptoms, there are a few points to consider.

For starters, not everyone who suffers from depression will exhibit each symptom on the list in the DSM. Some people will experience every single symptom, while others may only experience two or three. Secondly, the severity of these symptoms varies from person to person. Thirdly, how often a person will experience a symptom at any given time also depends on a lot of factors. There are biological, chemical, genetic, psychological, and social factors which come into play. There are too many variables to consider.

Because depression is a mental illness, it will actualize itself in different ways. Some people may become distant and reserved, while others might become outgoing and obnoxiously loud. Some people might stop eating while others will start stuffing their face. Even the same emotion can be manifested in different ways.

For me, 'anger' is shutting down completely. I have no patience for things which make me angry but I don't care enough to do anything about them. Frowning or shouting or throwing a tantrum requires effort. In fact, even writing about them is tiring. My anger is manifested as me retreating into my head completely and blocking out all external stimuli. I go on full autopilot mode (I'll explain this in a later chapter).

For others, 'anger' might be manifested as the stereotypical squinting and teeth-grinding, or starting a fight just so they have a reason to punch someone, or perhaps venting through the medium of poetry, or even playing GTA V and going on a rampage. It's very hard to explain the correlation between an action and an emotion, because human beings rarely experience emotions in isolation. We're constantly adrift in a sea of emotions. Trying to figure out what action is a result of which emotion is like trying to figure out where each drop of water in the sea originated.

Depression is horribly complex. My depression is probably completely different from what you're going through. The fog analogy I find so helpful might seem illogical to you. Maybe your depression is a tunnel which doesn't end. Maybe it's suffocating while everyone around you is fine. Maybe it's an excruciating numbness.

I am dealing with chronic depression, I've had multiple bouts of double depression in the past, and I probably will again. So if you're experiencing depression, regardless of what form it is, I can understand what you're going through because I'm going through something similar. But make no mistake, to say we're both going through the same depression is an insult to us and our daily battles against depression.

To defeat thy enemy, know thy enemy.

" Giving a phenomenon a label does not explain it. "

- Taylor Caldwell

Chapter Six

Pop Quiz, Hotshot

The language we use when talking about mental illnesses plays a huge role in how we perceive them. Stigmatizing language and vocabulary reinforces the misconceptions and stereotypes we have about mental illnesses. It's important to note that (most) people aren't using stigmatizing language on purpose. They're just ignorant on how it might affect the people around them.

Like a five year old with a label-maker, society wants to label everything. It doesn't matter if the labels are incorrect. We tend to talk about mental illnesses as though they're not a big deal. For example, if you like your items in a certain order, you've got OCD. (Actually, you've got CDO, which is the exact same thing, except the letters are in the right order.) If you drink a few cups of coffee, you've got ADHD. If you pull an all-nighter to revise for your exam, you've got insomnia. If you feel bad for failing your maths test, you've got severe clinical depression. If you think out loud while debating a particularly troubling issue, you've got schizophrenia.

Thinking like this makes light of the immense struggle people who are actually suffering from a mental illness have to go through on a daily basis. Society becomes desensitized to the importance of mental health. It's not that we're completely unaware of mental illnesses, it's just that we treat them with such a cavalier attitude that we're unable to take them seriously, even when we want to.

We can't see mental illnesses, so we don't think of them as being 'real' problems. We associate mental illnesses with quick fixes. *You've got OCD? Try not being so controlling all the time. You're depressed? Try being more positive in life.*

We treat physical problems differently because the disability is clearly visible and tangible. This helps people empathise better. *You've got a broken arm? I hope you get better! How did it happen?* We're quick to ignore how severe a mental illness is, just because we can't see how it manifests itself.

This stigma and ignorance rears its ugly head even when people are trying to be helpful. For example, when

I first found out I was suffering from depression, I was happy. I was finally aware that what I had been feeling for so long wasn't normal. Normal people didn't feel this way. There was something wrong with me.

It sounds weird, but knowing that I was somehow broken made me feel better. I didn't feel special or anything, I just felt pleased knowing that I had a problem. It gave me hope that I could solve the problem and actually get back to feeling normal. Whatever my normal was. (Cue Tylenol ad).

So I went online and researched depression. The websites I found at the time were all the same generic rubbish. I clicked on a link and I'd immediately be shown the vaguest possible list of symptoms. Aside from being frustratingly void of useful information, these symptoms could pretty much apply to every human being on the planet, depressed or otherwise.

These websites took a mind already wrought with doubts and self-loathing, and then shoved a massive list of contradictory statements in its (metaphorical) face. If you think I'm being harsh, one of the listed symptoms was that "You are sleeping too little". *Fair enough,* you might think. *Insomnia. That's a valid symptom.*

I would agree, except right underneath that statement, the other symptom of depression was that "You are sleeping too much". Really? I have never once in all my years on this earth heard anyone wake up one morning and say "Hey, you know what? I slept *exactly* the right amount last night!" Apart from Goldilocks, I suppose. But to be fair, she was eaten by bears, so it doesn't really count. (Also, she's fictional.)

If you're listing symptoms, you need to explain them properly. This is crucial. Hypersomnia and insomnia are two different symptoms of depression and they're not as simple as oversleeping and not sleeping enough. Listing them without any context or clarification makes it seem like you can experience both at the same time.

Obviously, lists like these are no substitution for a real doctor's diagnosis. The lists confuse people. They might as well replace the symptoms with things like "You go to sleep sometimes" or "You blink" for all the good it does.

Another really irritating thing is that a lot of websites say that two of the symptoms of depression are that you have difficulty making small decisions and that you often downplay/disregard your emotions. What would be the best way to approach an issue like this, where the very nature of the disease is that it skews your perception of self-worth and value?

I know! Let's create an unnecessarily long multiple choice quiz where each question has seven possible answers. Then, let's make sure each question is full of contradictory and confusing statements. This will really force the person to critically think about their emotions and thoughts. Depressed people don't have problems making small decisions, like you'd need to do for a multiple choice quiz, right? They don't have problems accurately assessing their self-worth and inherent value, right? Did anyone bother to research this? No? OK. It doesn't matter. I like this MCQ idea. Sounds like a solid plan!

If that's not bad enough, the questions on the multiple choice quiz are the *exact* same thing as the list of symptoms the website displayed just a few seconds ago. Seriously, all they do is take a symptom from the list and add a question mark at the end. Quite often, the questions don't even make any sense.

Of course you're going to be biased when you take the quiz. You're influenced by what you read, whether you notice it or not. Websites like these are unhelpful and lazy. Take the quiz and you end up with questions like this:

"Sleeping too much or too little?" *Yes.*

"Feelings of guilt?" *Yes.*

"Tired?" *Yes.*

"Numb?" *Yes.*

"RESULT: *It is possible that you could potentially perhaps maybe be a teeny tiny bit depressed, though I wouldn't really worry about it if I were you. You should sleep more. Also, you should sleep less. Have you tried not being tired?*"

I'm exaggerating (only a little), but you get the point. A multiple choice quiz is pointless, because your depression distorts your perception of reality. No matter what you choose, you're probably not going to get a completely accurate response.

You could be aware of your bias. You might try to pick something which you wouldn't pick, to accommodate for this. This sounds like a clever strategy, but it doesn't work. You end up with a result which doesn't apply to you at all because you went out of your way to pick the answers you think you wouldn't pick. Nobody is willing to answer 125 multiple choice questions twice, so instead of redoing the quiz, you try to convince yourself that the result you got fits you 100%.

These days, many of the websites which talk about depression are much better than the ones I first visited. But they are still not a substitute for a real doctor. Depression will wreak havoc with your brain and mental facilities. If you think you're depressed, even if you're not entirely sure, you need to talk to a medical professional. Do not rely on the internet.

An internet diagnosis a day keeps the doctor away.

" We can only see a short
distance ahead, but we
can see plenty there that
needs to be done. "

- Alan Turing

Chapter Seven

Zeno's To-Do List

Have you heard of Zeno's Paradox? If you have and you understand it, nice job. Head on down to the paragraph which starts with "That's the argument in a nutshell." I've bolded it so it's easier to find. Don't say I don't do anything for you. The rest of you, pay attention. I've broken the argument down in the paragraphs below.

Zeno of Elea was a Greek philosopher who wanted to show that motion is logically impossible. He came up with a bunch of paradoxes to illustrate how crazy it is that we're constantly in motion. Arguably, the most famous of these is the Dichotomy Paradox. Dichotomy literally means 'cutting in two'.

Imagine you need to travel a metre. Before you can travel a metre, you need to travel half the distance. Before you can travel half a metre, you need to travel a quarter of a metre. Before a quarter, an eighth. Before an eighth, a sixteenth, and so on. Before you can travel any distance, you must first travel half that distance. Each distance you need to travel will take a finite amount of time.

You can halve any distance an infinite number of times, which means that there must be an infinite number of distances you need to travel. According to Zeno, the only way to figure out how long it will take for you to travel the entire distance is by adding up the amount of time it takes to travel each distance. You might think that Zeno could just travel the distance and time himself like a normal human being, but unfortunately, he forgot his stopwatch at home. Obviously, this is the next best thing to do.

Zeno says that if you've split a distance into infinite pieces, and each distance has a finite time, then there must also be an infinite number of pieces of finite time. Travelling a metre (or any distance, for that matter) must therefore take an infinite amount of time, which is impossible. Therefore, Zeno concludes, all motion must be impossible.

That's the argument in a nutshell. The relevant bits, anyway. It's a fascinating read because it challenges our understanding of infinity and mathematics. We *know* that it isn't right; you can traverse a metre easily. It's hard to argue against Zeno's logic because at first blush, it seems weirdly true.

I bring up Zeno's Paradox because that's what depression has done to my brain. It takes something I inherently know is simple and easy to do, and amplifies it into a seemingly impossible series of tasks. The smallest of steps becomes an unclimbable mountain. It makes the most mundane of tasks too much for me to handle.

Imagine I need to brush my teeth, for example. Sounds simple enough. But before I can brush my teeth, I need to get to the bathroom. Before I can get to the bathroom, I need to leave my room. Before I can leave my room, I need to get out of bed, and so on.

Suddenly, brushing my teeth seems like a lot of work and effort. Too much work and effort. So I'll lie in bed, debating how important it is for me to brush my teeth. Is it worth the time and effort it will take? I ask myself the question for everything I need to do. For 99% of the scenarios I deal with, the answer is no. Very few things in life are worth the effort.

Deep down, part of me knows that brushing my teeth is not a lot of work. It knows that I can do it. I've done it loads of times before. It's easy. But that part of me is immediately silenced by the overwhelming voice that attacks me for being such a useless excuse for a human being that I can't even do something as simple as brushing my teeth.

I am worthless. Other people are getting on with their lives and I'm just sitting here unable to get out of bed. I am useless. My intuition is broken. I can never tell what the right decision is and I'm terrified of making the wrong decision because it would give my depression another reason to harass and humiliate me. Most days I end up doing nothing at all and I feel awful for doing so.

As you can imagine, this has affected my entire outlook on life. Life is one impossibly long to-do list. Every time I complete one task, another two are added to the list. The to-do list never ends. It's just chore after chore, task after task, responsibility after responsibility, obligation after obligation, until at last, I can die.

My depression constantly reminds me that other people are fine. Nobody else is having as much trouble deciding what to have for breakfast as I am. Life is easy for other people. Or at least they make it look easy. It's like they don't even know it's the hardest thing in the world. Why isn't life easy for me?

My depression constantly tells me that it's my fault. I must be doing something wrong. I'm a terrible excuse for a human being. I am useless. I begin to think that I'll never be able to be anything else. This is all I'll ever be. I will never amount to anything. This line of thinking stops be from livng. I no longer strive to be better. I am frozen in fear, steeped in doubt, and drifting alone in a sea of insecurities.

I'd end the chapter here, but it feels a bit too morbid a place to stop. So instead, how about I tell you how to solve Zeno's Paradox? The answer can be found through some simple calculus. Mathematically speaking, Zeno is talking about a convergent series. It's easier to understand it if you think about a square.

Imagine a square with an area of $1m^2$. Split that square into two equal pieces. If you split it into two triangles, don't. Stop trying to make things complicated. Just split it into two rectangles, like everyone else.

If you did it properly, you will have two rectangles with an area of $0.5m^2$ each. Take one of these rectangles and split it into two equal squares. Now you have two squares with an area of $0.25m^2$ each. Take one of these smaller squares and split it into two equal rectangles. You can continue doing this forever; you'll end up with an infinite number of pieces, each one smaller than the one before it.

If you calculate the area of each of these pieces and add them all together, you'll end up with 1m². You won't end up with infinity metres squared, because that makes no sense. Although there are an infinite number of pieces, each with a finite area, the area is getting smaller with each piece. The series converges (gets closer to a specific number) instead of getting bigger (what most people think of when they say infinity).

An infinite amount of time is not as simple as Zeno suggests. Let's say you and your female friend have plans for dinner. She phones you up and asks which restaurant the two of you will be eating in. You haven't eaten since breakfast. You check the map and realise that the closest restaurant is one metre away from your location. You know travelling a metre will not take an infinite amount of time because you understand Zeno's paradox.

Your friend wants to know if she should pick you up or if she should meet you at the restaurant. You tell your friend the restaurant's address, and tell her that you'll *metre* there. That moment, when you're chuckling at your witty joke and aren't sure if your friend is going to laugh with you or hang up the phone and never speak to you again, that is what an infinite amount of time feels like.

It feels like hunger.

" There is no more dreadful
punishment than a futile
and hopeless labour. "

- Albert Camus

- Chapter Eight -

Rock and Roll

The French philosopher, Albert Camus, has a blunt yet beautiful way with words. His most notable contribution to philosophy is the notion of the Absurd. The Absurd is the conflict between our desperate search for meaning in life and our inability to find it. We are trying to find some kind of purpose and value in a life which is devoid of both.

Absurdism is best explained through *The Myth of Sisyphus*. If you've not read the original version by Albert Camus, I'm going to paraphrase it in the paragraphs below. If you're one of the few people who actually has read the original, feel free to skip to the paragraph which starts with "Sisyphus is condemned to do a completely pointless task forever". I've bolded it for you so it's easier to find.

If you're going to ignore my suggestion and read through my paraphrased version anyway, I apologise in advance for completely butchering the original master-piece. The rest of you, ignore the previous sentence. My paraphrased version is 100% legit, okay?

Sisyphus is pretty much the original troll. This is a guy who would have sex with anything which moved, a guy who was probably on drugs all the time, a guy who would steal whatever he wanted whenever he wanted, just because he could. Sisyphus lived a very *rock and roll* life. If you don't get that awesome joke, don't worry. It'll make sense in a few paragraphs.

Sisyphus was a genius who loved life. He hated death. A lot. One day, Sisyphus decided to kidnap Death (a.k.a Thanatos, the god of death) and lock him up in the base-ment, just for the hell of it. Because that's just the kind of guy Sisyphus was. He held Death prisoner and then went on with his life like everything was fine. All around the world, people who were supposed to die just carried on living.

As you can imagine, this was a pretty nasty situation. A decapitated person, or a person who died of old age, or a person who died of dysentery would just be walking around like everything's fine. Ares, the god of war, got annoyed that nobody was dying in any of the wars he incited. Ares freed Death from his chains and told him where Sisyphus was hanging out.

Needless to say, Death was furious at being imprisoned. The second he got out, he went to kill Sisyphus for being an arrogant jerk. Death dragged Sisyphus to the Underworld. Sisyphus, of course, had planned for this.

Sisyphus told his wife to mess up the burial rites. When a person died, it was customary to place a coin in their mouth before you buried them. The coin, known as Charon's obol, was meant as a payment for Charon, the ferryman who transfers souls from the land of the living to the land of the dead. Sisyphus's wife 'forgot' to bury Sisyphus with a coin in his mouth and she didn't observe any of the other burial rites either.

When Sisyphus finally got to the Underworld, he couldn't pay the ferryman. Feigning annoyance at his wife for messing his burial up, Sisyphus asked the guy if he could go back to life and berate his wife for being incompetent. Charon, who probably didn't get paid enough to deal with this kind of stuff, let Sisyphus go. Sisyphus was given three days to get his affairs in order before he would have to get back to the Underworld.

Of course, Sisyphus had no intention of going back. He stayed on Earth for years and eventually died of old age. The gods got seriously peeved at being tricked twice by Sisyphus so when he finally showed up in the Underworld, they sentenced him to an eternal punishment.

Every single day, he would have to push a gigantic boulder - a gigantic *rock* - up a huge mountain. When Sisyphus got to the top, the boulder would *roll* back down, and Sisyphus would be forced to push it back up again. Over and over again. For all eternity. Because the gods seriously know how to hold a grudge.

Sisyphus is condemned to do a completely pointless task forever. That's exactly what a depressed person thinks of life; a series of pointless obligations until you die. Camus says Sisyphus represents humanity; we love life, hate death, and are forced to do something pointless for all eternity. We're searching for the meaning of life, even though we'll never be able to find it.

Sisyphus is aware of his condition. The gods probably gloated about the punishment, and Sisyphus is using it against them. He is revolting. Not that he's disgusting or anything (though the hygienic system at the time was terrible). He is rebelling against his eternal punishment. Sisyphus has embraced the absurd, pointless nature of his punishment and is defying it. He has learned to love the struggle itself. The gods wanted to punish him by making him do a completely pointless task, but if he's enjoying the task then it kind of ruins the fun for them. That is his small rebellion.

Sisyphus has accepted that his life is pointless, so he's stopped hoping for something better. In doing so, he no longer views his punishment as a punishment. It is simply his life now. That is what makes Sisyphus the absurd hero. He has embraced his punishment. He has stopped trying to think of his life as having some profound meaning or destiny. He has come to terms with the fact that his life is what it is. Nothing more. Nothing less.

In the same way, Camus says we should embrace the absurdity of our lives. We should acknowledge that life is chaotic and without meaning. It isn't the result of some god's grand plan. There is no purpose to it. It is pointless.

Camus says that embracing the absurd nature of life doesn't mean we should commit suicide. Just because we realise that there is no point to life doesn't mean we should kill ourselves. Instead, Camus says we should revolt.

We should continue to search. We should defy the idea that we'll never find meaning. Accepting our absurd reality gives us the power to create and assign meaning to things as we deem fit. Think of it like this: there's no point to making watch if nobody is going to use it to tell the time. It serves no purpose until we assign one to it and use it the way that we want to.

The only way to truly be happy is to accept the fact that your life is your own. Just because there's no purpose to life doesn't mean that your life is pointless. You must create your own meaning, your own purpose, your own worth. You must embrace your life and learn to love it for what it is. Love the good parts and love the bad parts. Be your own absurd hero.

My depression and I are the two parts of the Absurd. I'd love for my life to have any semblance of meaning or value. I'm desperately searching for some purpose I can build my life around. My depression, on the other hand, tells me that I'm wasting my time. Life is not worth living. It's pointless exertion until I die. It is meaningless.

The idea of a meaningless existence terrifies me. I'm afraid of having to wake up every single day and continue living for no reason whatsoever. The only good thing I can see is my death; my meaningless life will one day be over. At least my pointless existence isn't eternal. Immortality would be awful.

I want my life to have meaning but I'm struggling to create it myself. How do I figure out what is meaningful when my depression is trying to convince me that nothing is? I don't want to spend my life doing something based solely on the hope that it'll all pan out in the end. I need a guarantee. I need facts. I need proof.

Imagine you spend ten years studying for a test you can only take once. You show up on the day of the test and find out that you had been studying the wrong subject. Despite your best efforts, you did the wrong thing and you failed. Ten years of wasted effort, even though you believed you were studying the right thing. It would crush you.

I live with that fear and guilt every single day. I know I need to give my life meaning and I feel guilty for not doing it. I can't do it because my depression has drained me of the ability to recognise value. I am dead inside. I look around and see nothing which is meaningful to me. Life is just the thing I'm forced to do while I wait for death.

It's paralysing. I am trapped in this fogging nightmare. I can't take a single step in any direction because I will never be able to know if that step is in the right direction. I am lost. I am disoriented.

There is no way out.

" I grow numb; I grow stiff. How shall I break up this numbness which discredits my sympathetic heart? "

- Virginia Woolf

Chapter Nine

Autopilot

I've always thought of my brain as a separate entity to myself. I am the incorporeal half (the mind or soul). My brain is the corporeal half. We're controlling the same body, but we're each in charge of different things. There are things which I do (the stuff I'm actively and consciously doing/thinking) and then there are things which my brain does (things like keeping my heart beating or maintaining a proper breathing cycle).

My body, which is an entity separate to me and my brain, is just a physical thing. It's literally just a vehicle which transports me and my brain. And a pretty pathetic vehicle, at that. It hates moving, it whines when it doesn't get enough sleep, it starts making weird noises when it hasn't been fed for a while, and it's got a completely random waste disposal system.

I think, or at least I hope, that most of you can relate. We always think of ourselves as a mind in a body. It's like when you hit your foot on the coffee table. You don't immediately think, "Me!" You think, "My foot!" And then you probably hop around the living room, shouting obscenities at every piece of furniture, thinking that they were all in on this ambush together.

I find this incredibly fascinating. Not the whole furniture-planning-to-destroy-humanity idea (although that would make a decent Michael Bay movie with explosions and absolutely no storyline or character development whatsoever), but the idea that we can't escape duality. Whether it's mind and body, good and evil, right and wrong, or light and darkness, duality is intricately connected to humanity. I'm adding another element to the mind-body duality, which means that we're dealing with three things: me (the mind/soul), my brain, and my body.

I am always in the driver's seat and I control the body's active actions; things like telling my body how to move or what to say. My brain takes care of the subconscious stuff; the things I can't or don't actively control, like remembering to blink or properly digesting food. (Except now that I've just written down the whole 'blinking' thing, I've become aware of how often I blink. Control of that particular bodily function temporarily belongs to me until I forget about it, at which point my brain takes control of it again.)

Every now and then, I get tired of being in charge of my body's active actions. It's exhausting. That's when I switch to autopilot mode (I let my brain take over for a while). Autopilot is great because it lets me live in my head without having to worry about dealing with the external world. I apologise if the analogy is getting complicated, so let me try to make it easier. Here's a breakdown of how autopilot works.

1.   My body is like a car.

2.   I am in the driver's seat. I am controlling the active actions of my body. I tell my body where to go, what actions to do, what things to say etc.

3.   My brain is in the passenger seat. It is controlling the subconscious actions of my body. It tells my eyes to blink, my heart to beat, my lungs to breathe etc.

4.   At the same time, my brain (being a supremely talented multitasker) observes how I drive. It looks at how I react to certain situations, what fa-

cial expressions I tell my body to make, how I tell my body to move, what things I tell my body to say and when to say them etc.

5.   Whenever I get tired of driving, my brain will jump into the driver's seat and take over. Even though it's now in charge of the active actions of my body, my brain still continues to control the subconscious actions of my body. It does both jobs very well.

6.   Meanwhile, I will be in the passenger seat, doing literally nothing at all. I'm no longer in charge of anything my body does. I have no responsibility. It feels amazing. I am free.

7.   Of course, I'll occasionally glance at the driver to see if everything's running well. My brain's almost got his full driving license now, I'm so proud!

8.   It's important to remember that this is all happening inside my head. On the outside, nobody will know anything's different. Because my brain is so good at pretending to be me, it will control my body exactly like I would.

For example, imagine I'm at dinner and the discussion turns to the political situation in Canada. Bored, I will be busy wondering if fish actually *do* have fingers they're not telling us about. My brain notices this, agrees that fish are hiding things from us (I never trusted them), and automatically takes over control of my body.

It tells my body how to act. It makes all the required facial expressions and even throws in a few insightful comments to convince people I am really listening to the conversation. To the outside world, nothing has changed. Internally, I'm not paying the slightest attention. I have no idea what people are saying. I have no idea what my brain-controlled body is saying. I have no idea of anything that's happening in the real/external world, because I can't be bothered to care.

I go on autopilot quite frequently, because real life is nowhere near as interesting as the stuff which happens in my head. I go on autopilot mode when I want to skip parts of my life. It's a refined form of daydreaming. It's sort of like sleeping; you close your eyes at 9:00 p.m. and when you open them again, it's 7:00 a.m. You've just skipped ten boring hours of your life.

Autopilot is my fast-forward button for life. For example, I get on the bus to go to university. The next thing

I know, I'm already sitting in the lecture hall and have even written up a few notes. I've no idea what happened in between these two events, but I'm sure it was boring. Otherwise I wouldn't have gone on autopilot.

I switch to autopilot when I'm commuting, when I'm watching a boring TV show or movie and the remote is too far away for me to change the channel without getting up, when I'm not focussing on whatever I'm reading, or even when I'm talking to someone. Apparently, I've had multiple conversations while being on autopilot.

Although I'm a big fan of autopilot, I always switch back and get in the driver's seat again. I feel safer, knowing that I'm (somewhat) in control of my body's actions. But ever since I encountered depression, I've lost that feeling of security.

If you've ever driven in dense fog, you know what I'm talking about. You have to drive very slowly, you've got to check your mirrors every few seconds, and you become more self-aware than ever. You become paranoid that you might make a mistake and crash. Depression amplifies these doubts and fears until your self-confidence is completely shattered.

Every second I drive, it tells me I'm about to crash. It plays all the mistakes I've made in the past and reminds me that I'm a terrible driver. It screams that I'm not strong enough to deal with the responsibility of driving a car. It tells me I should just give up driving. I mean, it's obvious that I'm rubbish at it.

In fact, my depression whispers that I should crash my car on purpose, just so that I will no longer be a danger to anyone else. *A pre-emptive safety measure*, it tells me. *Just drive off the cliff and it will be safer for all the other drivers on the road. You're a hazard to other people. You're a terrible accident just waiting to happen. They'll be better off if you weren't here. Just drive off the cliff.*

I become paralysed by the fear of hurting other people because of my inability to control the vehicle. Like the spineless coward I am, I tell my brain to take over indefinitely. I shift over to the passenger seat, secretly relieved that I'm no longer in control. I don't deserve to be in charge of my life. I'm not strong enough to deal with all that responsibility.

At this point, my car is surrounded by the fog. The fog is so thick, it's somehow gotten into my car. It has created a soundproof barrier between me and my brain. I watch as depression manipulates and violates my brain. I can see what it does, but I'm powerless to stop it. I can see what my fogged up brain tells my body to do, but I have no say in the matter. My brain, being a brain, is not aware of the fog.

Much like proper mind control, my brain has no idea it's being acted upon by an external force. As the autopilot protocols dictate, it carries on driving like it normally would. So when people ask me how I'm feeling or what life is like, my brain will tell my body to say "I'm fine. How about you?"

I think most people would be freaking out at this point, because they have absolutely no control of their life. But strangely, I think of it as a kind of liberty. I find myself not caring what happens to my body because I'm no longer responsible for it. I am free.

I realise this line of thinking might be strange, but I haven't even gotten to the really weird bit yet. Putting up a facade and pretending that I'm fine is easier than baring my soul and telling people I'm dealing with depression, intrusive thoughts, crippling social anxiety, and perpetual existential dread.

Most people don't know how to deal with that. If I tell them, they'd just feel bad for me, and I would end up feeling bad for making them feel bad. Everyone's got their own problems to deal with. Their lives are probably hard enough without me dumping my troubles on them. I have no right to burden them with something I should be able to handle myself.

Furthermore, (and this is the bit which is properly weird) I'm not 100% sure depression is even a problem. Like I mentioned in a previous chapter, I feel like I need my depression. I know that I'm thinking this because depression has skewed my perception of reality. But for some reason I don't mind the fog. It's what I know. I'm used to it. It's familiar. It's reassuring. It has become my comfort-zone. It's coated me in a layer of apathy. Apathy is freedom from consequence and responsibility.

Depression has made me numb and indifferent to most things. I'm completely detached from my own reality. It's like I'm watching a TV show of my life, but I'm somehow not even the main character. And it's not even a good TV show. I'm only watching because I can't change the channel. It never hits me that this is a show about my life. This detachment is evident in even the most trivial of moments.

For example, a person holds the door open for me. I watch as my brain tells my body to do something. My head moves up and down. I feel my face twisting. Is it a smile? I can't tell. I don't care. I see the person frown and ask me if I'm alright. My brain tells my body to do something else. I feel my mouth move as I tell the person I'm fine. My face contorts into what I can only imagine is a friendly smile. The person smiles confusedly and walks away. The moment passes. Life goes on.

It's like I've become a zombie or a robot with a broken circuit board. My body is just going through the motions, acting like everything's normal, because that's the only thing my brain knows how to do. I didn't prepare it for driving in the fog. In all honesty, I didn't expect that I would even run into fog. Like I said before, you never really notice depression fogging up your life until it's too late.

Let's go back to the point about facades and keeping up appearances, so I can explain the rationale behind that particular line of thinking. This book is meant to show you how depression messes with a person's head. I know that bottling up my thoughts and emotions isn't a particularly healthy way to deal with depression, but depression convinced me otherwise.

First off, everyone has problems in their lives. They are capable of dealing with their problems. That's what humans do. Pretty much every motivational speech in the world will have a bit about how we can overcome the hurdles in our life if we put our mind to it. I see people struggling with the problems in their lives every single day. Their problems are often worse than mine.

So depression has made me apathetic. So it tells me my life is not worth living. So it convinces me that I'm a burden to everyone around me. So it tells me I should kill myself. So what? Do I really have a right to complain about my problems? There are people in the world who don't have access to clean drinking water, or food, or shelter. There are people who have lost friends and family members because of bombs and shootings and religious fanatics. There are people who were forced to watch the new Fantastic Four movie in its entirety because they had to review it on their blogs.

Compared to all these people and their real problems, my life is amazing. I've got a loving family, great friends, a wonderful house, more food than I need, constant electricity, clean running water, and I've not watched the new Fantastic Four movie. I am blessed. I have no right to feel bad about my problems.

If anything, I should be grateful that I've got depression. It could be worse. I might have cancer or AIDS. I should be grateful for all the things I have, and I should be grateful for all the things I don't. I have no right to feel upset.

At this point, I feel bad for feeling upset, because my depression has convinced me that I have no right to that emotional response. I have no right to feel upset, so why am I feeling upset? My depression convinces me I should be punished for feeling upset instead of being grateful for all the good things in my life.

I'm unable to argue with my depression's logic; my life is great, what right do I have to feel bad? (This is where it gets super-confusing.) I'm supposed to feel happy for not feeling bad (my life could have been a lot worse), but at the same time, I'm supposed to feel bad for not feeling happy *enough*. My depression punishes me for being depressed. My depression punishes me because according to it, I have no reason to be depressed. Do you see how backwards that logic is?

In my fogged up head, it makes perfect sense. This is how perfectly depression manipulates people. Not only does it torture me emotionally, but it actually makes me *want* to torture myself, just so I have a reason to justify my emotional response to life. It convinces me I deserve this eternal punishment and then hands me the torture kit. I become the victim and the torturer at the same time.

And I can't tell myself to stop.

" When we are tired, we
are attacked by ideas we
conquered long ago. "

- Friedrich Nietzsche

Chapter Ten

Megaphone

When I was going through a period of Major Depression, I found myself wishing that I wasn't alive anymore. I would go to bed at night hoping that I wouldn't wake up in the morning. My life was just an endless stream of pointless misdirected effort. Day after day, as I forced myself to go through the motions of life for reasons I couldn't fathom, I couldn't stop thinking about how life would be so much easier if I wasn't alive.

The thought had been fairly dormant in the back of my mind for quite some time, ever since I first dealt with chronic depression. I was dimly aware of it floating around and mumbling just out of earshot (if my mind had ears), but it had never been loud enough for me to pay it any attention. It was simply a silhouette in the fog. But when

I was going through a major depressive episode, my depression found that thought and handed it a megaphone.

My first strategy was to try to ignore the thought, but that quickly proved impossible. That megaphone-wielding thought was the only thing I could hear in my head. My second strategy was that of an exasperated parent; if my depression and I couldn't learn to share the thought-space in my head, then neither of us could have it. I tried to not think any thoughts at all.

I don't mean I tried yoga or found spiritual enlightenment or nirvana or anything like that. I mean I would binge-watch TV shows so mind-numbingly stupid, I could feel my IQ dropping. I mean listening to music at a volume so loud that it would drown out every rational (and irrational) thought in my head. I mean forcing myself to stay up for days at a time so that I would get so mentally exhausted that other irrational thoughts would pop up and fight with the megaphone-wielding one for supremacy.

Of course, these were short-term solutions to a long-term problem. And they were pretty stupid solutions. Everything I did just made me tired. And when I was tired, that megaphone-wielding thought would get louder and louder. It was exhausting trying to think of anything other than not wanting to be alive. The moment I tried, my depression would just turn the volume up on the megaphone.

It was like trying to start a conversation with someone in the front row at a concert. The only way you're going to manage a halfway decent conversation is if you start shouting at each other. And that's going to annoy the band, so they'll start playing louder, which causes you to shout louder, which causes them to play louder. And it's a cycle of stupidity until your throat is sore, your head hurts, and you realise your conversation wasn't worth the effort anyway.

If I had the capacity to care at the time, I would have been frustrated beyond belief that I could think of nothing else but not wanting to live. I mean, how pathetic do I have to be to not even be able to control the thoughts in my head? Instead of frustration, I was intrigued by the notion of not being alive anymore. Compared to my predicament at the time, it felt like a pretty welcome alternative. I should clarify here that I was not, am not, and never have been suicidal.

Let's use the "Life is a rollercoaster" analogy everyone uses. Imagine there are two people sitting on the rollercoaster and both of them are sick of the ride. Both of them want the same thing; to get off the ride. The suicidal person would jump off because that is the only viable option he sees. The wanting-to-not-be-alive person (let's call him Bob) wishes he had never gotten on the ride in the first place.

That's the difference. That's what I felt. I've experienced the ride and it was fun for a bit, but I'm done now and I want to get off as quickly and safely as possible. Of course, there were other reasons why suicide wasn't the right choice.

First off, suicide is expressly forbidden in Islam. Even if I wanted to kill myself, I wouldn't do it because it goes against everything I believe in. Secondly, the desire to not be alive is not the same as the desire to commit suicide. There's a subtle but important difference between the two. It's like the infamous philosophical Trolley Problem.

Imagine a trolley is hurtling towards five people tied to a track. You're standing next to a lever which will force the trolley on to a different set of tracks, where a single person (let's call him Bob) is tied to tracks. If you do nothing, the trolley will continue on its course and those five people will die. If you switch the tracks, you kill Bob. Do you let five people die or do you kill Bob?

In response to this question, most people turn into utilitarians. They argue that the best thing to do is that which brings about the greatest possible good for the greatest number of people. In other words, utilitarians argue you should switch the tracks, reasoning that one death is better than (not as bad as) five deaths.

There's a very important thing to note here. People want to switch the tracks *because they want to save five lives*. Nobody wants to switch the tracks because they want kill Bob. Well, nobody apart from that one guy who tied Bob to the tracks in the first place. Whether you switch the tracks because you hate Bob or because you want to save five people, the end result is the same. It's the *intention* behind your choice which makes all the difference.

It's the same thing when it comes to not wanting to exist anymore. I wanted to not be alive, but that doesn't mean I wanted to commit suicide. If there were a way to not exist without going through the whole dying process, I would pick that in a heartbeat.

Not wanting to be alive felt like the right choice. Depression is death's waiting room. You go through the motions of life, even though you know it's meaningless, because you're just waiting to die. Life is temporary. Only death is permanent. I was already emotionally, physically, and spiritually dead. I was just waiting for my mind to kick the bucket and then I'd be on my way. I was existing, not living. I felt that I was a burden on other people. And I had decided that it would be better for me, my family, and my friends if I wasn't around anymore. The only problem in my plan was that dying takes effort.

If you think you're a burden now, just think about what happens when you die. Your family will have to arrange the funeral service, someone will have to dig the grave, someone will have to move your body from wherever you end up dying (and let's face it, nobody dies in a convenient place) to a more suitable location, they'll need to clean your body, and people will have to take time out of their day to come to your funeral, if they even decide to show up.

Your family and friends will grieve for a very long time and generally feel terrible about the whole ordeal. They'll have to get rid of all your stuff and learn to live without you. Given time, you will fall away into obscurity and be nothing but a memory. And a poorly reconstructed one, at that. Sadly, the human brain isn't very good at retaining accurate memories.

Not existing, on the other hand, is awesome. The best part about not existing is that it's quick and painless. I'm assuming it's quick and painless, of course. Obviously, since I'm writing this and you're reading this, neither of us have managed to figure out how to not exist yet. But you get the point.

If you never existed, you wouldn't have to worry about anything. Your family and friends wouldn't mourn or grieve or even miss you, *because you were never a part of their lives*. You wouldn't be a burden on anyone. You wouldn't cause any negative emotions or pain. You would be nothing at all. Of course, since you don't exist, there wouldn't really be a 'you', but let's not overthink this.

You might argue that I would never get to experience happiness or hope or love or anything good. My response would be that I wouldn't have to experience sadness or regret or hatred or anything bad. And I'm willing to give up every good thing in my life if it guarantees I will never experience any terrible things.

I was obsessed with the idea of not existing. I tried discussing it with a few people, but it's kind of hard to bring it up in everyday conversation. Death, depression, and suicide aren't really things people enjoy talking about. Murder, on the other hand, is fine, for some reason. Mass murders are an even better topic of conversation.

But the moment you bring up depression and death, people get squeamish. They'll either laugh it off and try to change the subject or they'll overreact and call every emergency number known to man, convinced that you're literally going to drop dead in the next five seconds. There's no simple way to talk about it.

You can't walk up to your friend and say "Hey, so I've been thinking, wouldn't it be cool if I wasn't alive? Non-existence would be awesome, amirite? Why are you backing away? Is it because I said 'amirite'? How could you even tell? This was a purely verbal conversation! Wait, did you just dial 911? I'm not suicidal!"

And then you spend the rest of the conversation consoling the person and convincing them that you're not suicidal and that you know life is worth living and that you'll never scare them like that again and that it was just a hypothetical question and that of course you'll never think about death in the future. Once they calm down, you know you can never talk to them about your depression again because they'll probably freak out and you're just not emotionally equipped to deal with all their feelings. With that knowledge, a part of you dies inside. Your isolation/alienation becomes that much more real.

People also react weirdly when you try to be direct. When I tell people that literally the only reason I wake up is so that I can go back to sleep or that I sometimes wish I never woke up at all, they awkwardly smile and assume I'm joking. They tell me I've got a twisted sense of humour and then rush off to continue doing whatever they were doing before I bothered them with my existential crisis.

That being said, I did manage to have a really long and in-depth conversation with a close friend of mine (Let's call him Bob). One day, we decided to skip our lectures and go to the university library instead, so that we could properly discuss everything. After roughly six hours of discussing life, death, good, and evil, we somehow ended up talking about how easy it would be for Santa Claus to take over the world with an army of dentists.

I can't remember which one of us won the debate (it was probably Bob), but I distinctly remember thinking that it was one of the best discussions I've had in a long time. It was great because there was no judgement. Bob didn't start pre-emptively spewing solutions to my potential problems and nor did he just sit there and agree with me like some sycophantic suck-up. There was no molly-coddling or sugar-coating or fear that if he said the wrong thing I might just off myself. Bob talked to me like a rational human being and it was an honest, open discussion. It managed to kill the voice in my head.

For a while, at least.

A few months later, I got the news that after a long and painful fight with cancer, Bob had passed away. Just like that, one of the most genuine and intelligent people I had ever met was gone. As I came to terms with the loss, the thought sprung back to life and I was once again plagued with the idea that life would be better if I didn't exist.

Fast-forward a year or so, and now I'm sitting here, writing this book with the hopes that I've done at least a mediocre job at explaining what goes on in a not-suicidal depressed person's mind. Also, I've come to terms with the fact that there's absolutely no chance of me figuring out how to not-exist without dying or killing myself.

I've therefore decided that, much like the rest of my life, following that particular train of thought is a complete waste of effort. Instead, I should focus my energy on something less pointless. It's not a particularly happy notion, but it keeps me going. Of course, the thought of not wanting to exist still pervades my mind, but on the plus side, it's no longer as loud as it was.

I think the battery on the megaphone might be dying.

" Man alone measures time. Man alone chimes the hour. And, because of this, man alone suffers a paralyzing fear that no other creature endures. A fear of time running out. "

- Mitch Albom,
The Time Keeper

Chapter Eleven

The Nervous System

Fear and anxiety are two different things. Fear is your brain's reaction to a real, immediate, objective threat. Imagine you're walking home at night and a guy pulls a gun out, demanding your wallet. Your brain is going to panic because the threat is very real. That is fear.

Anxiety produces the same physical response as fear. The only difference is that anxiety is not the result of an immediate or apparent threat. Your brain can't figure out where the threat is coming from but is convinced that the threat is real and it reacts accordingly.

Imagine you're standing on the top of the Burj Khalifa, peering down at the streets of Dubai. You lose your balance. There's a split-second where your life flashes before your eyes, your heart beats so fast it feels like it'll burst, your stomach does backflips, your eyes water, your head pounds, and you don't know if you're going to fall backwards or regain your balance. You're teetering on the edge of the unknown and it induces a horribly uncomfortable anxiety. Imagine you feel that way *all the time*. That's what it's like to deal with anxiety.

I'm eternally agitated. I'm uncomfortable in my own skin. I feel like I've forgotten to do something really important and I can't remember what it is. I am constantly worried, but I don't know why. It's an inescapable, ineffable, unstoppable anxiety, scratching away at the inside of my head.

It's very difficult to translate this anxiety into words because I don't even know what I'm afraid of. Anxiety is fear of an objectless threat. All I know is that I'm filled with dread. I have an unshakeable feeling that something bad is going to happen, and when it does, I will be powerless to stop it.

I've talked about this in previous chapters, but I'm terrified of doing nothing with my time. I've got a horrible feeling that my life is some kind of cruel existential joke. I can either spend my life finding my true purpose, or I can spend my life fulfilling my true purpose. The sick twist is that I only have enough time to do one of these things.

I can't fulfil my true purpose in life if I never figure out what it is. But at the same time, it doesn't make sense to search for my true purpose if I know I'll never be able to fulfil it. Either way, I lose. This fear, that my time is running out before I can figure out what to do with it, is known as chronophobia.

Chronophobia is the fear of time. It's the fear of time moving too quickly or too slowly. It's the fear that your time is running out. It comes from the Greek word "chronos", meaning time, and "phobos", meaning fear.

The etymology of the word doesn't really capture the feeling itself. I don't think chronophobia is just the fear of time passing. I think it's the fear of time without meaning. Time without purpose. Time without value. It's the fear that you're wasting your time.

I feel like a colossal failure because I haven't figured out what to do with my life while everyone else is getting on with theirs. It bothers me that other people make it look so easy. People my age are getting married and starting companies and maturing into functioning members of society, while I'm stuck in the same place, emotionally and mentally. (Probably physically too, since I haven't left my house in weeks).

My mind is so fogged up, my intuition is broken. I can't tell what the right thing to do is. I'm paralysed by the fear of making yet another mistake. I'm afraid to take a single step because for all I know, I might be stepping in the wrong direction. My time is limited and I don't have the luxury of making mistakes.

Time is a rope slipping through my fingers. The more I freak out about how quickly it's slipping, the tighter I grip on the rope, in the hopes that I'll be able to slow it down somehow. But the tighter I grip, the more my hands get cut. So I'm forced to let go. Then I freak out about how quickly the rope is slipping through my fingers and the cycle starts anew.

This fear pervades every waking moment of my life. It pops up in the tiniest and stupidest ways. I mean really stupid ways. For example, I can't watch movies anymore. I can only watch TV shows. Why? Because I can't commit to wasting two hours of my life watching a movie. It's a completely illogical, irrational, stupid reason not to watch movies. *Especially* because it is stopping me from rewatching the extended editions of the Lord of the Rings movies.

I'm fine with binge-watching TV, but I feel a sense of dread when I look at the running time of any movie. My heart pounds and my knees feel weak. I start to hyperventilate. It's ridiculous to feel this way. It makes no sense.

I'm no psychologist, but I assume it's because a part of me feels relieved that I can stop watching whenever I want. I don't have to make a long-term commitment. It's like reading a 10,000 page book. I'm more likely to read the book if it's divided into small chapters instead of having no chapters at all. I feel a sense of security, knowing I don't have to read the entire book in one go. I can stop whenever I want. I have multiple escape routes.

I have escape routes in real life, too. Before I even walk into a building, I need to know where the bathrooms and emergency exits are. I get anxious in wide open spaces because there's no place for me to hide. Wherever I am, I need to know that there is a place where I can escape and hide. Even if I never use it, I just need to know that it's there. I feel safer knowing that it exists.

I've developed the superpower of being able to rationalise and justify any decision I make because of my anxiety. I haven't been to university in three weeks. I make up excuses to justify my actions. Stupid, random, illogical reasons which somehow make sense to me. Just last week I rationalised my decision not to go to a very important lecture because it was raining and I could have slipped and shattered my hip and people would have laughed at me. It makes no sense.

I can forgive the shortness of breath, the clammy hands, the chills, the throbbing in my head, the watering eyes, and even the waves of nauseating pressure which flow from my head right down to my toes, but I cannot forgive the fact that this anxiety makes no sense to me. It serves no purpose and follows no logic. It just shows up, freaks me out, and then leaves. I'd be able to better deal with this anxiety if I knew why it happens.

I worry about stupid things. Whenever I sit, I try not to cross my legs because I worry that I might twist them so much my kneecaps might pop off. I constantly grit my teeth because I worry that my teeth will fall out at any moment, so I have to push them back into my gums. I don't like using tin-cutters because I'm afraid that I'll cut the top off and it'll slice my eyeball. I don't like driving because I worry that I might one day listen to the voice which tells me to ram my car into the nearest obstacle. I panic when I hear a loud noise because I worry my eardrums will start bleeding.

My fears are affecting my morality. I think I am becoming a less morally good human being. For example, one of the things I try to do on a regular basis is help other people. I think we can all can agree that helping others is a morally good thing to do.

I used to help people because I thought it was the right thing to do. That was enough for me to do good deeds. But now, my intentions have changed. I don't help other people because I'm an inherently good person or because helping others is its own reward or because I'm empathetic. I help other people because it distracts me from my own life. By focussing on their problems, I temporarily forget about my own anxieties. I use other people for my own selfish reasons.

To the other person, my intentions make no difference. Whether I help them because I'm a good person or I help them because I need a distraction, the end result (for them) is the same; they get helped by me. But the motivations behind my decision are ultimately selfish.

I'm so selfish that I genuinely do not even care about the other person or their problems. I have become completely apathetic. I no longer see people as people. I only see them as a means to an end. They're just things I use to distract myself from my troubles. My best friend could get shot in the face right in front of me and the only thing I would feel is annoyance at the fact that I lost my distraction and have to find a new one. This apathy disturbs me.

As disturbing as it is, this apathy only seems to block out the positive aspects of my thought process. It will easily block out empathy, hope, kindness, and happiness. But it lets my depression roam free. I am emotionally numb but I retain my moral knowledge. My depression will take any immoral thought or action I have, even if they're against my will (like the selfish apathy), and use it prove to me that I'm a terrible person. I feel less than human. I am afraid of myself.

In many cases, fear is a great motivator. People procrastinate because the impending deadline forces them to work. Getting work done in a caffeine-induced, last-minute scramble is what people (students especially) seem to enjoy. Fear forces us to jump into action.

Because of my depression, fear doesn't motivate me. I am numb. Fear doesn't inspire me to make the most of life's experiences while I have the chance. I haven't travelled the world or learnt a bunch of languages or made a friend named Bob or cherished every day on this Earth as if it were my last. All I've done is worry and have panic attacks while I hating myself for being who I am.

I can't focus on my work. I can't focus on my hobbies. I have trouble falling asleep because I stay up every night and think about all the time I wasted that day. Then, the next day I think about all the time I wasted while lying in bed thinking about all the time I wasted during the day; I could have done something worthwhile with all that extra time if I wasn't going to spend any of it sleeping.

I am using this book as an opportunity to be as open with you about my mental illness as I can. But with every word I write, I can feel my depression or anxiety or whatever the hell it is in the back of my head start to panic and worry that it's not good enough. I worry that people will read this book, criticise it, and judge me for being a whiny, self-indulgent, chronically insecure, boring person.

I'm trying to break down my walls and show you the real me, so you can understand just how badly depression and anxiety mess with a person's mind. But in doing so, I feel exposed and vulnerable. I feel the need to build new walls to protect myself from your judgement and criticism.

I know this book could be better written and I will forever hate myself for being unable to express myself properly through writing. Language is as much a bridge to clarity as it is a barrier. In any case, I am baring my soul to you in the hopes that you can use it as a conversation piece to talk about mental health.

I also want to say that if you think you've got an anxiety disorder or if you think you're suffering from a mental illness, you should talk to someone. Nobody should have to live like this.

You deserve a better life, even if you don't believe that you do.

" Blessed are they who
see beautiful things in
humble places where
other people see nothing. "

- Camille Pissarro

- Chapter Twelve -

Beauty in the Beast

For most of this book, I've been treating depression like the perfect unbeatable villain. And that's misleading. I've beaten it before. I've gotten past multiple major depressive episodes. I'm still here. I persist. I will not go down easily.

I've realised that if I'm going to beat depression permanently, I have to stop romanticizing it. I need to treat it like a realistic enemy. I'm not a superhero and depression is not a supervillain. It's just a part of my existence.

Depression is not perfect. It fluctuates. It falters. It loses. Yes, there are days where I want to not be alive, but there are also days where I'm productive. Days where I get things done. Days where I appreciate the good things in my life. Days where I temporarily fight off the fog and spend a few hours basking in the sun.

As I mentioned in an earlier chapter, we can find duality in everything. Depression is no different. I want to get rid of the fog because I hate it, but I also like it because it's become comfortable for me. Fog can be disorienting and frightening, but it also has a surreal sense of beauty.

And the beauty of depression is that it has made me actively *want* to be a better human being. It's broken me down completely. It has pushed me to my limits. It has shown me the worst parts of myself. And that's a good thing. I look at all the darkness inside of me and through it, I can see the light. As Martin Luther King Jr. once said, "Only in the darkness can you see the stars."

Let me say right now that this chapter will not resonate with everyone, especially those who are still very much in the depths of their depression. I know you might be thinking that there is nothing good at all about depression and you're right. Depression sucks.

But for me to beat depression, I need to accept that it played a role in making me who I am today. I can't ignore its positive aspects and focus solely on its negatives. I have to find the balance. For all the bad days I've had, I've had a few good days as well. This chapter is a reminder to myself that there is always good, no matter how small, in the bad. I just need to look hard enough. These are the positive things I learned from my depression.

1. I'M LESS JUDGEMENTAL

I understand that I'm not the only person dealing with a problem. If I've hidden my problems for so long, it's possible that others might be doing the same. I used to judge other people based solely on their actions while I justified my own actions on my intentions. Everyone in life is going through a struggle I know nothing about, so I have no right to pass judgement on anyone. All I can do is be kind.

2. I'M MORE EMPATHETIC

This goes hand in hand with the first point. My life sucks and I'm hiding it from the world. (Yes, the best way to hide a mental illness is to write and publish a book about it.) I've learned that I'm not alone in my struggle. Through my depression induced late-night Googling, I realised that there are thousands of other people who are suffering from depression.

And that thought is strangely motivating. Nobody should have to feel like this. If you're suffering from depression, I genuinely want to help you get through this, because I know what it's like. I wouldn't wish depression on my worst enemy. You're in a dark place right now, but if I can be a light for you, even for a second, then that's what I want to do. We're in this together.

3. I'M NOT AFRAID OF DEATH

This is both a good thing and a bad thing. I'm not afraid of death because I welcome it. Death is a lot of things, but the main thing I focus on is that it's permanent. Sleeping is great, but I know that I'll eventually have to wake up again. That simple fact ruins my sleep. With death, you sleep forever. And that sounds pretty great from where I'm at right now.

Again, just to clarify, I don't want to kill myself and I don't suggest you do either. I just don't want to be alive anymore. I won't say I'd jump out the way if a car were about to run me over, but I also won't go out of my way to dive in front of cars and intentionally get run over either. There's a very slight difference there, but it matters to me.

4.   I Don't Get Embarrassed

During the early years of my depression, it mattered a lot to me what other people thought. I was terrified of going out because I knew everyone was secretly judging me on my appearance and my body language and the way I spoke and about a hundred other reasons. My depression convinced me that my entire life was some kind of The Truman Show situation, where everyone was secretly in on the joke apart from me.

But my depression has gotten to such a stage that I don't give a rat's fart what other people think of me now. I've got enough problems to deal with without pretending that I'm psychic and know what everyone is thinking. Unless someone (let's call him Bob) comes up to me and actually tells me he thinks I'm stupid and worthless, I'll just assume everyone's minds are as vacuous and empty as my emotional capacity. Not a nice thought, but it keeps me from being so self-conscious all the time.

5.   I Think Critically

This is probably a result of me overthinking everything. It's not something I'm actively doing, but my depression forces me to think about every possibility in life (and how each one is going to be terrible). My thought process goes through some rigorous parsing before I'm happy with what I've thought of. Most things in life aren't worth the effort so if I'm going to spend my time thinking about stuff, I better be sure it's worth it.

6.   I'm More Appreciative

If I can get out of bed today, then that's a big deal for me. It reminds me that depression is not permanent. The little victories are everything. Every now and then, the fog dissipates and the sun comes out. The sunlight may be fleeting, but I sure as hell appreciate it that much more.

7.   I Am In Touch With My Emotions

Thanks in part to chronophobia, I'm fixated on the idea that I need to be the best possible person I can be. This means I have to be better mentally, spiritually, physically, and emotionally. That last one was always a problem for me. Even before my depression, I had trouble expressing my emotions.

Being a male doesn't help. There's stigma associated with masculinity; that 'real men' don't let their emotions out. If I go up to another man and say anything remotely emotional, the standard response is to assume I'm being weird.

I realise now that not being able to let your emotions play out can drastically exacerbate and elongate depressive swings. Depression has locked up all my emotions but left me things like Guilt and Shame and Self-Loathing. I'm pretty good at those. It's the other ones I need to work on. Happiness, Hope, Pride, Courage, and Sadness, to name a few.

The fact that my emotions are locked up is actually helpful. I'm not bombarded with a rush of emotions which would completely throw me off. Every now and then, an emotion escapes from its prison and I experience it in isolation. It might sound weird, but I feel happy to feel sad. Much like Point #6, I don't get to experience emotions much, so when the odd one shows up, I appreciate it a lot more than I normally would.

8.   I'M AN EXCELLENT LIAR

This one is self-evident. I don't mean to brag, but I've managed to hide a mental illness from everyone in my life for years. Nobody in my life has any idea what kind of person I actually am. Depression wants me to feel alone and the best way to do that is by being surrounded by people who will never know the true me. I pretend that I'm fine and nobody can tell that I'm dead and empty inside.

9.   I'M HUMBLER

I know, I know. Just by putting this on the list, I'm exemplifying an ironic lack of humility. Because depression has totally shattered my perception of self-worth, I will forever underestimate myself. I will always sell myself short. I will disregard every positive thing about me and instantly believe the negative things about me. I'm not sure if it's humility or a complete lack of self-esteem, but

I'm putting it on the list anyway because it makes me feel better.

I know I've essentially listed nine positive aspects of depression, but you will never hear me say that depression is a good thing. It's like getting both your hands cut off but saying that at least you don't have to cut your fingernails anymore. Depression sucks. I wouldn't wish it on my worst enemy.

But finding something good about depression has somehow made it weaker. It has allowed me to externalise my depression. I am finally seeing my depression as something which isn't a part of me or my identity. In listing its positive aspects, I've found its weak-points. (I was toying with the idea of making an Achilles' heel reference because it fits perfectly with the whole Greek mythology thing I've got going on in this book, but it might get too confusing.) I am finally seeing that glimmer of sunlight breaking through the fog.

I think this is what Hope feels like.

66 We rise by lifting others. "

- Robert Ingersoll

Chapter Thirteen

Could You Not?

It's impossible for someone who's never experienced depression to truly understand what it's like. When I first found out about depression, I Googled the hell out of it. I came across hundreds of websites about the mental illness and I was quite pleased that so many people were talking about it.

Then I noticed that for every website which talked about the seriousness of the issue, there were about twenty which would post some ridiculous listicle thing which would focus on the "Top 10 Worst Things to Say to Someone Suffering from Depression" or something equally inane.

The worst thing about these kind of posts is not that they're useless and bereft of helpful information. The worst thing about these websites (and also Buzzfeed) is that it's because of them we've ended up with the word 'listicle'. It's either a list or an article. Not both. Stop making stupid words. Not everything needs to be blended. (And yes, that is the correct linguistic term for when you combine bits of words together to make a new one).

But to get back to the point of these posts being useless, the list on each website has the same ten points listed in different orders. The general "Top 10 Worst Things to Say to Someone Suffering from Depression" list will usually look something like this:

1. Just snap out of it!

2. Have you tried not being depressed?

3. What reasons do you have for being depressed?

4. At least it's not as bad as...

5. Are you sure you're depressed? You seem OK today.

6. It's all in your head.

7. It'll all be OK in the end.

8. I know exactly how you feel.

9. Just exercise more!

10. Think of all the people who love you!

I browsed through a few of these websites, naively thinking they might offer some advice on how to talk about an issue as important as depression. *They'll list the bad stuff to say and then will tell me the good things to say, right?* Nope. Instead of advice, these websites were spewing passive-aggressive, sarcastic rubbish aimed at shaming non-depressed people for not knowing what depression is like.

As you can imagine, this annoyed me quite a lot. A lot of these people have popular blogs, best-selling books, or a fairly active YouTube account with loads of subscribers. They've got a platform for their voice to be heard by hundreds of people. Instead of doing something good with it, instead of raising awareness about a serious mental illness, instead of giving advice on how to deal with depression, these people think that the best thing to do with their time is to put non-depressed people on a guilt trip for not knowing how to properly talk about depression.

These blog posts are useless. They make non-depressed feel guilty and angry at being attacked for no reason whatsoever. The lists make depressed people feel even worse about themselves because it further isolates them by creating an intangible barrier between them and non-depressed people. These websites make ridiculous generalizations that every single person experiences depression the same way, which we know isn't true.

So what if someone said one of the things from the list? At least they're making the effort to talk about depression. I understand that depression is not a fun topic of conversation, but that doesn't mean we should attack people for not saying the 'right' thing. People who care about us want to help. We shouldn't ostracize them because they don't know how to.

If you're suffering from depression, focus on the fact that people who care about you want to help you. Right now, you might even think that no one cares about you. As impossible as it may seem, I want you to ignore that thought. It is lying to you.

Of course there are people who care about you. Focus on them. It'll take a lot of time, but use that as your foundation and then take baby steps from there. It's a team effort; you need to help them help you. It's going to be tough and awkward, but this is a conversation which needs to happen.

If you're not suffering from depression, please understand that depression makes people cut themselves off from society. It's alienating. It's isolating. It's frightening. It'll take time for a person suffering from depression to become comfortable enough to talk about it. The most important thing you can do is provide constant support. I don't mean you should be repetitively asking them if they're OK and mollycoddling them, but just let them know that you'll always be there if they need help.

Just knowing that there were people looking out for me and checking in on me from time to time did wonders for my self-esteem. For this final chapter, I've outlined the things which other people said/did which helped me out when I was going through a double depression.

Obviously, this is my personal experience and I can't guarantee that this approach will work for everyone. I can't say that what I'm experiencing is how everyone will experience depression. I can't say that what helps me deal with it is going to help others as well. But these are the things which helped me and I hope you find some of them useful.

First of all, the most important thing is to not treat a person suffering from depression differently. One of the main reasons I didn't want to talk about depression was because I knew people would instantly see me in a different light, like I've got a gigantic FRAGILE sticker plastered across my face. It's the exact opposite of that stereotypical scene in any romance movie where a girl fixes her hair and suddenly everyone realises she was super-attractive all along.

Depression is stigmatised in that people often think those who suffer from depression are emotionally or physically weak. This is complete and utter rubbish. Depression doesn't care if you're strong or weak or old or young or male or female. It will latch on to you for absolutely no reason and then work on killing you from the inside. It has nothing to do with weakness. The fact that you wake up every single day, knowing that you'll have to deal with depression again, is a testament to your perseverance and strength.

So if you want to talk about depression, don't treat the depressed person any differently. Don't mollycoddle them, don't baby them, don't sugar-coat things. Don't treat them like a fragile thing which could break at any moment. Talk openly and honestly. Again, this might not work for everyone, but it worked for me.

I will always prefer the truth over a lie, even if you're lying to spare my feelings. If I tell you I am depressed, don't tell me what you think I want to hear. Talk to me sincerely and openly. If you've never experienced depression, don't say something like "I know exactly how you feel!" because I know that you don't. (I know this is one of the things from the list, but I'm not going to insult/berate you if you say it to me. I'm only using it to explain why I find it annoying and unhelpful.)

As I mentioned in a previous chapter, I don't have access to all my emotions. As a result, my mind will focus on the literal content of a message instead of the emotions behind it or the manner in which it was said. I will focus on the literal aspect of language rather than the more abstract/metaphorical stuff. I'm doing a horrendous job of explaining why I think this way, but that's just how my mind operates.

Feel free to say things like "I can only imagine how you must feel!" Saying something like that tells me you're being honest. It also shows me that you're trying to empathise with my current predicament. It shows me you realise the gravity of the situation. You're not lying to me and I appreciate it.

On the flip side, if you're going to lie to me, do a good job of it. Make sure I never find out. There is nothing worse than a sloppy liar. If I find out you've been lying to me, even if it was about a trivial thing, then we're done. You've lost my trust and you're probably not going to earn it back again. From that point on, I will never be able to tell if you're telling me the truth or if you're lying to me. That doubt will always be in my mind whenever we talk, and it's just easier for me to assume that every word out of your mouth is a lie. Trust and fidelity are very important to me. Respect that.

Secondly, and this point stems from the first point, when I talk to you about my depression, I need it to be in a judgement-free zone. Even if you don't act on your judgement by treating me differently, please don't secretly judge me. I know this sounds stupid, because I will never be able to know what you're secretly thinking, but still. Remember that I am still the same person I was before my mental illness, I'm just in a very dark place right now. I'm already thinking that you're judging me and it would kill me if I found out my depression-induced suspicions were true.

Not judging others is something I'm still learning how to do, but I realise now how important it is. When I was diagnosed with depression, my first instinct was to hide it from the rest of the world because I knew they'd judge me if I told them. It's easier to put up a facade and pretend everything's OK, because that's what everyone else does with their problems.

I didn't talk about my depression for about eight years. Mainly because I didn't know how to bring it up in casual conversation and also because it was my problem and mine alone. I didn't want to burden other people with my issues. In hindsight, that was a terrible perspective to have. I was depressed, alienated, and terrified of people finding out about my secret. I was in a very dark place.

So if I do talk to you about my depression, leave your misconceptions, judgements, and stigma at the door. I'm feeling very emotionally exposed and vulnerable. I feel bad for bringing it up because I know you'll feel pity for me or you'll feel bad for not knowing how to help me. It really helps if you ask questions and seem interested and ready to talk about depression. It makes me feel that you're comfortable talking about this stuff and you're not doing it just to make me feel better.

Thirdly, it's OK if you're not sure how to deal with a depressed person. If you've agreed not to judge me, then I've no right to judge you either. It took me eight years to become comfortable to talk about depression. This is your first time, it's OK if you make mistakes or say the wrong thing. As long as you don't pretend that you know how to deal with a depressed person, we should be good. Depression is definitely a tough conversational topic, but I'm glad that you're here with me, even if our conversations are full of pregnant pauses and awkward waffling.

Fourthly, our conversations don't always have to be so serious. This won't resonate with everyone, but I think humour, terrible jokes and awkward humour especially, can be a great way to deal with depression. Acknowledging the awkwardness of the situation can make it less awkward.

For example, when I first talked to a friend of mine (let's call him Bob) about depression, he made the stupidest joke. I can't recall the whole conversation but I remember there was a point where I told him that I'm depressed. Bob instantly replied "Hi, depressed. I'm Bob."

Bob had the goofiest grin on his face, like he was actually proud of his 'wit'. It was a terrible joke, but it was the perfect ice-breaker. I felt completely at ease, discussing mental health with him. I know some people might be appalled at the levity with which we were talking about such a delicate issue, but depression doesn't need to be a serious issue. Humour makes it better. Don't be afraid of making stupid jokes. The stupider the better.

Fifthly, be patient and don't take things personally. I know that I've severed many a relationship and pushed people away because I've been apathetic, rude, and insensitive. I did not (and often still don't) care what you say. I know that sounds rude, but that's just the way I think. If you tell me it'll all be OK in the end, I'll probably reply with some sarcastic remark about you being a rubbish fortune-teller and wanting my money back.

I will be rude to you and I will say some inappropriate things because I'm just venting. Don't take it personally. I'm trying to push you away because part of me believes that you're going to leave me anyway. It's the difference between getting fired and quitting. I want to push you away but I also want you to stay with me until the bitter end. It's a weird thing, wanting two completely different things at the same time.

I push you away because I think it'll be better for you. When I die, I won't burden you with grief, since we will not be friends by that point. In my fogged up head, I'm doing you a favour. You deserve a better friend than me. I'm apathetic, I'm lazy, I'm rude, I'm sarcastic, I'm boring, and I'm insensitive to your needs. Yes, I am suffering from depression, but that doesn't give me a free-pass to be mean to everyone else in the world.

If you're willing to stick with me regardless of what I'm forced to be when I'm depressed, then I will love you for it. I know it's asking a lot. I tend to get annoyed and irritated at myself for just existing, so I can imagine how much of a burden I must be to other people when I'm severely depressed. But if you can just be patient long enough that I get past this, then you are an impossibly good person and I'm lucky to have you in my life. Continue being awesome.

Sixthly, we don't always have to talk about depression. This links back to the first point; don't treat me differently. Send me a message and ask me if I want to get dinner later. Talk about what you did on your weekend. Complain about how bad that Fantastic Four movie was. Don't predicate every conversation with a head-tilt accompanied with the usual "Are you OK?" I don't want every conversation we have to be related to depression. It's probably as annoying for me as it is for you.

Just act normally. You've done more than enough for me. It's time I do something for you. (Well, I say it's for you, but it's mainly for me. It helps me if I can pretend to be a normal human being for a while. It's a nice change of pace from the daily self-loathing.) If I need to talk about depression again, I'll bring it up. You've shown me you're open to talk about it without passing any judgement on me, so I will be comfortable enough to talk to you if ever I need to. Thank you.

Seventhly, don't give me solutions. Not to sound rude or arrogant, but the chances that you'll be able to suggest something which I haven't come up with in the past nine years, especially knowing that you don't know much about depression, is very slim. I am talking to you just to vent my anger at depression. I want you to nod angrily and say "Yeah!" or "You're right!" or even the odd "Depression must suck!"

Please don't pre-emptively start throwing out solutions to a problem you don't fully understand. I don't quite understand it myself and I've dealt with it for nine years. Don't get overly emotional either. The worst thing for me is when people unload their emotions on me. I have very few emotions these days that I'm just not emotionally equipped to deal with all of yours. It's exhausting and physically draining when I have to console you.

Of course, that doesn't mean I don't feel obligated to reciprocate. You're listening to me complain about my issues, so I will try to do the same for you. I can't put into words how much effort it takes to deal with all the different emotions people have. It's like a blind man seeing for the first time. It's overwhelming. The best thing for both of us is to keep our emotions in check.

I understand that your solutions are coming from a good place. You genuinely want to help me and it's nice of you to think out loud and voice potential solutions to my problem. You might even think it's good to approach the problem with an optimistic outlook. Don't. Just don't.

I know you're trying to help, but because of my depression, I will find your positivity and hope annoying. I find happy people irritating beyond belief. I don't know why. I will think you're naïve. I will assume you're lying to yourself, because you wouldn't know true happiness if it slapped you in the face. Maybe it will get better. Maybe it won't. But your hope is useless. I have no need for it. Keep it to yourself.

I'm just here to vent. You're just here to listen. I don't need solutions. I don't need you to solve the problem. I just want to you agree that the problem sucks. I realise that you might think that repeating a platitude to me might be helpful. It's not.

It just trivialises the whole issue. If I could solve depression by understanding that "it's all in my head," then I'd have done it by now. Also, side-point; it's not all in my head. Depression has physical symptoms too. It causes aches and pains in places I didn't even know I had.

I know I keep going back to this, but the most important thing you can do is to not treat a depressed person differently. I know it's really weird not knowing what to say or how to deal with what's happening, but the fact that you're trying is good enough. Trust yourself to just be with them in the unknown. They'll appreciate it more than they can ever express.

Hopefully, this book shed some light on the fogged up mental illness that is depression. I hope it showed depressed people that they're not alone. I hope that it showed non-depressed people what it's like to deal with depression.

I know this isn't a story of success or a particularly happy book. But I truly do want to help you fight depression and rid the world of stigma. Use this book as a platform. Use it to reach out to people in your life, even if it's just to vent. You could say something like "This Zaeem guy, what a pretentious git! I bet he doesn't even have any friends named Bob! This guy doesn't know anything about depression. Depression is a fog? Yeah, right. Depression is ...."

See what you've just done? You've opened up to people about your depression. You've made it the topic of conversation without making that conversation awkward or uncomfortable. That is progress, my friend!

Also, it'll make the other person want to buy and read this book (don't give them your copy), just to see how bad it is. Recommend this book to people who care about you or people who are going through a tough time. The stuff I talk about in this book can be used as a conversation starter your friends and family can use as catalysts to reach out to you. We can beat this fogged up mental illness if we work together. We can defeat depression. We *will* defeat depression.

Depression doesn't get to win.

" Alone we can do so little;
together we can do so
much. **"**

- Helen Keller

Acknowledgements

Although my name is the only one on the cover, the production of this book would not have been possible without the help and support of several key people.

First and foremost, I will forever be grateful to my parents, Muhammad and Sajida, and my siblings, Areesha and Ali, for their unwavering support and eternal encouragement.

A sincere thank you to Professor Guy Allen for giving me complete creative control over the entire book-writing process and for guiding me along the way.

I thank Ali, my loyal copy-editor, who was forced to print multiple copies of my manuscript and go through them all with a ballpoint pen in one hand and a dwindling supply of caffeine in the other.

Omer Tahir and Syed Hamza Ali also get a special mention for their invaluable feedback and constructive criticism. If it weren't for our thought-provoking late-night discussions about depression and mental health, I would have gotten a lot more sleep. Thanks for that. I hope you're happy.

Lastly, my dear reader, I would like to thank you. Thank you for trusting me with your time. Thank you for fighting to rid the world of stigma. You are awesome.

And you know what?

So am I.

" Knowing yourself is the beginning of all wisdom. "

- Aristotle

About the Author

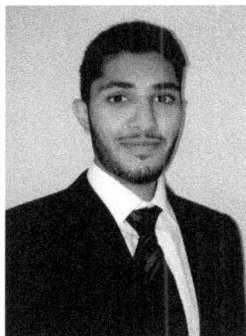

ZAEEM SIDDIQUI is a part-time writer, perpetual procrastinator, and full-time introvert who constantly seems to find himself in socially awkward situations. Born and raised in the UK, Zaeem is now living in Canada, after a brief stint in the deserts of Saudi Arabia. When he's not busy contemplating the meaning of life, Zaeem's hobbies include updating his blog (Introvert@Uni), reviewing gadgets on YouTube, and running away from his responsibilities. In his spare time, he makes fun of terrible movies and geeks out over obscure Doctor Who references. He doesn't have any friends named Bob.